AF800796

Rykerr Medical's

Vent Management Guide

for Invasive Mechanical Ventilation in Transport

Version 1
May 2020

RYKERR MEDICAL LLC

Legal Statement

Rykerr Medical LLC presents all of this good stuff for education purposes only. While we hope that the content here will be of use to our audience in the clinical setting, all actions taken by consumers of this information is at the discretion of the individual and should be in accordance with organizational policies, professional scope of practice, appropriate medical direction, and/ or current best practice. We have done our best to provide references for all ideas not our own and to utilize sources that are both truthful and reputable.

RYKERR MEDICAL LLC

Rykerr Medical's

Vent Management Guide

for Invasive Mechanical Ventilation in Transport

Table of Contents

EMT – emergency medical technician; **NM** – New Mexico; **OK** – alright; **QR** – quick reference; **SpO$_2$** – pulse oximetry

A Personal Intro

There are a lot of good reasons why I thought it'd be good to put together a primer on vent management, but the main one is that my first vent experience was a near-disaster and I'd like to share what I've learned since then so that others can avoid what I had to go through. I also think there's some room for diversity in how we, as an industry, present material to each other and move forward with our understanding of complicated things. And lastly, I hope is that this interactive style of writing can be of help to some folks and maybe inspire others to do the same and build on the whole idea. Collaborating together to improve our skills and holding one another accountable to live that out through clinical practice means better care for more people.

But to start with the awful beginning story: I was brand new to an ambulance service in New Mexico, having moved from Pittsburgh about two years after I first got my medic. I was still green but felt like I had gotten a lot of experience back in the city and was maybe a tad over-confident. Anyway, I started at this rural service in mid-November and the call that prompted my journey down this path of ventilator self-education was the day after Thanksgiving. I had basically just arrived in NM, barely gotten settled into the second EMS service I had ever been given medical control at, and was turned loose to practice in the field.

Things were different for sure. Five- and ten-minute transport times had been replaced by ones that sometimes took hours. With a five thousand square mile coverage area, the ambulances were giant machines that could be rigged to carry three patients each and would never have made it in the city alleys. Protocols and capabilities were a lot more lenient and included vents, surgical crics, hiking to patients broken in the woods - that sort of thing that this city boy just hadn't done before.

Oh, and also two-patient interfacility transfers. Our flagship hospital was in Albuquerque, one hundred and eighty miles or two and a half hours away by bus, so it was hugely advantageous to load two patients in on a single truck to avoid and extra six-ish hours of that second truck being gone from the service area. And when I was asked if I was OK with a vent patient and a psych patient going up to Albuquerque at the same time I didn't turn it down and we started getting things together. Part of that prep process was another guy showing this guy how to use the LTV1200, as I hadn't gotten to that part in my orientation and didn't yet have the confidence to say "no" to things I wasn't comfortable with or ready for.

My five-minute vent lesson was subpar, to say the least, and then I was off to the big city with the vent guy on the stretcher and the psych guy on the bench seat, two EMTs up front just in case I needed anything. My first action when the vent started beeping was to press that handy silence button – per the lesson I had received on the machine's operation. When that didn't work I figured it might be because the patient wasn't listening to the vent settings we had dialed in before leaving, so I paralyzed him – also per the lesson I had received. And that worked for a little while. Then I started getting more alarms and a low sat, so I did what all good medics do and disconnected the vent, grabbed my BVM and had the EMTs up front pull over so that one of them could hop in the back and give me a hand.

Sats stayed low, the alarms were yelling at me, the EMT was like, "come on, bro, get it together," and I didn't know what to do. So I turned the vent off, pulled the tube out, and started over from the very beginning with BLS airways and the BVM. That happened, we had the airway secured, sats came up, and then I handed the bag off to the EMT and set my sights on restarting this vent machine the way I had been taught just a little while ago. It was during this process that I realized my connections from the machine to the circuit had come undone. I must have stepped on them or something during the shuffle… Nowadays I would have simply looked at which alarm I was getting and worked through a systematic process for addressing it. The whole fiasco would have been avoided. But back then I didn't know a single thing about vents, to include that the text on the screen was relevant to getting the alarm to stop.

BLS – basic life support; **BVM** – bag valve mask; **DVD** – digital disk storage; **$EtCO_2$** – end-tidal carbon dioxide; **EMS** – emergency medical services

And that's just part of the story. One other part, don't forget, is that guy on the bench seat watching the whole damn thing and me hoping he stays cool enough that I don't have to try and manage two patients simultaneously. Another part is that even though I finally did get that alarm situation sorted, I still had trouble managing my vent settings. I couldn't maximize my SpO_2 or keep my $EtCO_2$ in range, my patient would get super agitated every time the Vec wore off, etc.... We did, however and finally, arrive to the big city in a presentable state – perfusion was good, sats weren't embarrassing, the patient appeared comfortable enough and was making some effort to breathe on his own, and that machine had stopped yelling alarms at me.

With the patient handoff complete, I returned back to small town New Mexico late on that day after Thanksgiving, year 2012, and decided then and there that I was never, ever, going to be in that situation again. My initial study list looked something like this:

The Ventilator Book by William Owens

The LTV1200 Product Manual (and the DVDs)

EMCrit Dominating the Vent Series
Part 1, Part 2

I later came across many other great resources and I will mention those as we get to them. And also, I got on the technology train. Which I think is a huge facilitator of learning when used in the right way and I hope that this little experiment can demonstrate that. In this print version of the manual you can just scan the QR codes for any of the references to access them (if available for free) or to see where you can purchase them (if they want your money); if you want an electronic version (for free!), visit us at rykerrmedical.com or follow the QR code on the title page to link to the website.

So now let's jump into the weeds and see where we end up. Keep in mind that this is to be an ongoing project and my first foray into this type of thing – so if you have feedback, just send it my way or offer to lend a hand. I'd love to get more folks involved in this and to make it both better and more accessible for everyone.

PEEP – positive end-expiratory pressure; **PPV** – positive-pressure ventilation; **PCO_2** – partial pressure of carbon dioxide; **PO_2** – partial pressure of oxygen

Some Very Basic Physiology

Before discussing mechanical ventilation, we need to cover fundamental concepts of the respiratory system and the breathing process. The stuff outlined here is intended only to give a foundation for understanding vent management. One recommendation for looking into the details beyond this (much of which comes up later when we talk about specific conditions) is a good, solid, heavy Anatomy and Physiology textbook or any of the references noted.[1]

The Normal Breathing Process

Let's start with a picture of what major components we are working with in normal inhalation and exhalation. At its most basic, we have the lungs and the large airways:

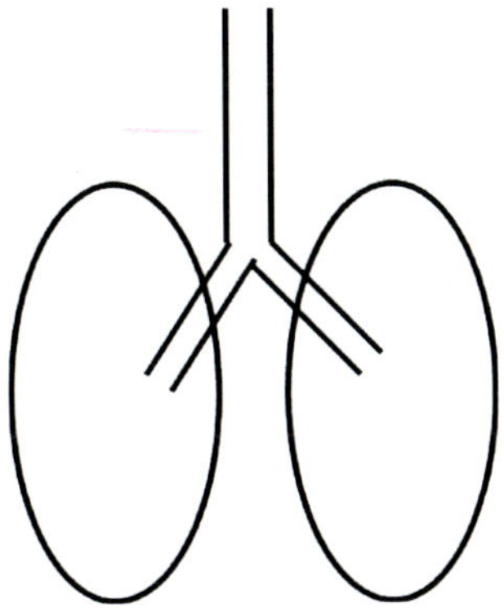

We also have the chest cavity and the diaphragm:

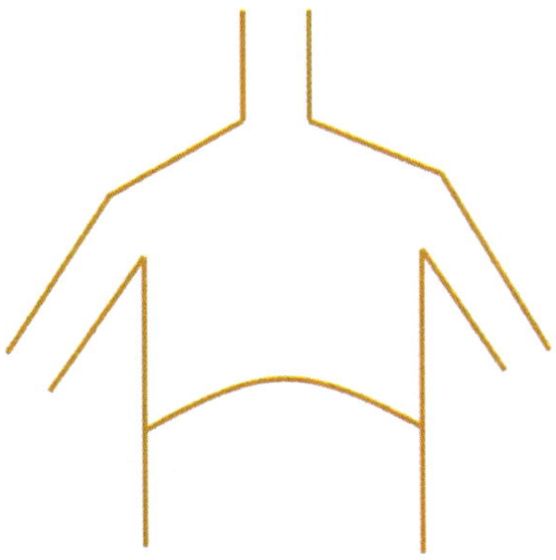

[1] Also see **Suggestions for Further Study** at the end for more content on both vent management and the physiology behind it

ARDS – acute respiratory distress syndrome; **cmH_2O** – centimeters of water; **CO_2** – carbon dioxide; **mmHg** – millimeters of mercury
O_2 – oxygen; **OK** – alright

The lungs are attached to the chest cavity and diaphragm so that when the diaphragm contracts or flattens, the lungs expand – this sucks air into the pleural space via a negative pressure:

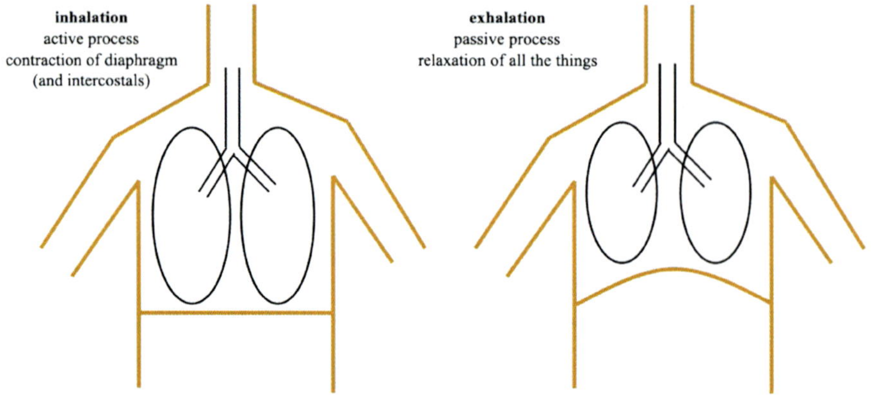

Inside this same cavity lie the heart and great vessels; most important to our discussion is the inferior vena cava:

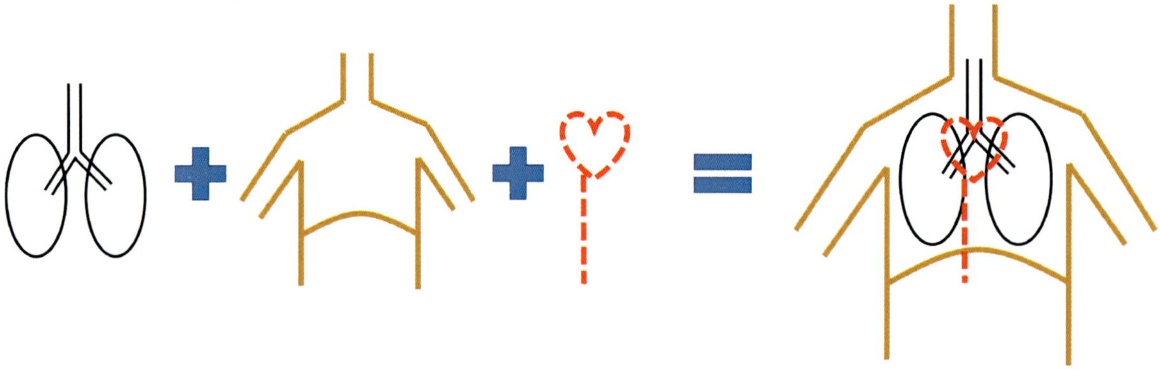

We have a system that normally functions by contraction of the diaphragm (with or without help from the intercostal muscles) to create a negative pressure, sucking of air into the lungs.[2] Because this air movement occurs via negative pressure, blood return via the inferior vena cava is facilitated by normal ventilation.[3] This will be important when we move on to talk about positive-pressure ventilation in just a minute.

---

[2] Hasudungan, 2014 – To review the physiology of breathing in a bit more detail, refer to this video
[3] Azizov, 2017 – Another video that explains the mechanism by which normal breathing supports cardiovascular processes

PEEP – positive end-expiratory pressure; **PPV** – positive-pressure ventilation; **PCO_2** – partial pressure of carbon dioxide; **PO_2** – partial pressure of oxygen

Zooming in, the image below shows blood vessels encircling little sacs, known as alveoli, which are the homestay of pulmonary gas exchange where oxygen (O_2) goes into the blood and carbon dioxide (CO_2) goes out:[4]

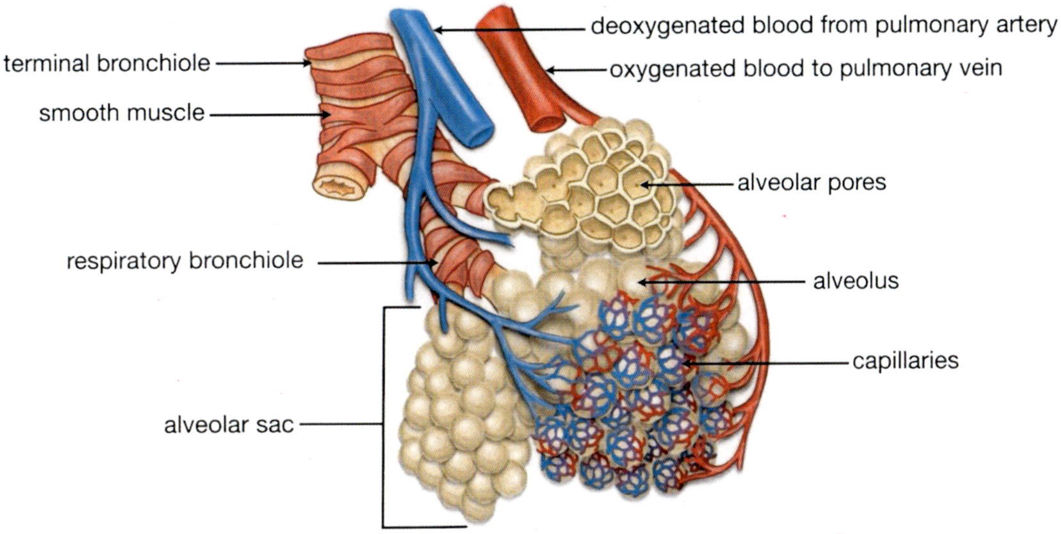

A simplified version of a single alveoli with a corresponding blood supply can help us understand the pathophysiology of different situations:

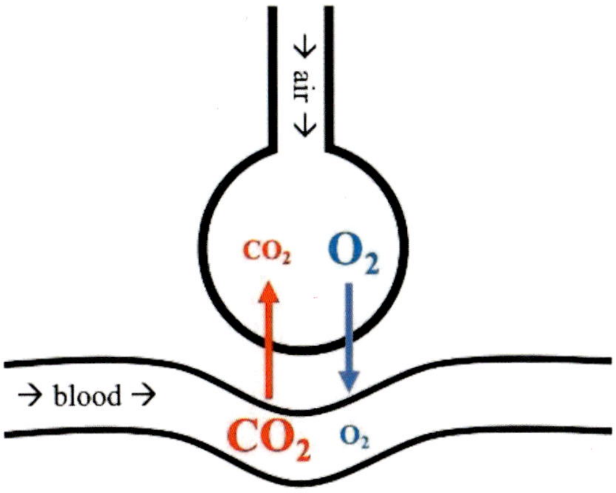

[4] Graphic built by Dr. Sameer of *Art by Dr. Sam* on Fiverr and *The Young Orthopod* on YouTube

ARDS – acute respiratory distress syndrome; **cmH₂O** – centimeters of water; **CO₂** – carbon dioxide; **mmHg** – millimeters of mercury
O₂ – oxygen; **OK** – alright

Next, let's add some numbers to that graphic of a single alveoli and its blood supply.[5] Note that in real life blood is continually moving past the alveoli and gases are constantly shifting to reach equilibrium, so that as carbon dioxide is offloaded and oxygen is onloaded, there is a new supply of blood and a reset of the gradients across that membrane. Plus the diffusion of gasses from alveoli to pulmonary capillaries happens very quickly. This means we generally aren't worried about this timeframe (i.e. how fast these gasses diffuse) being the limiting factor in this process:[6]

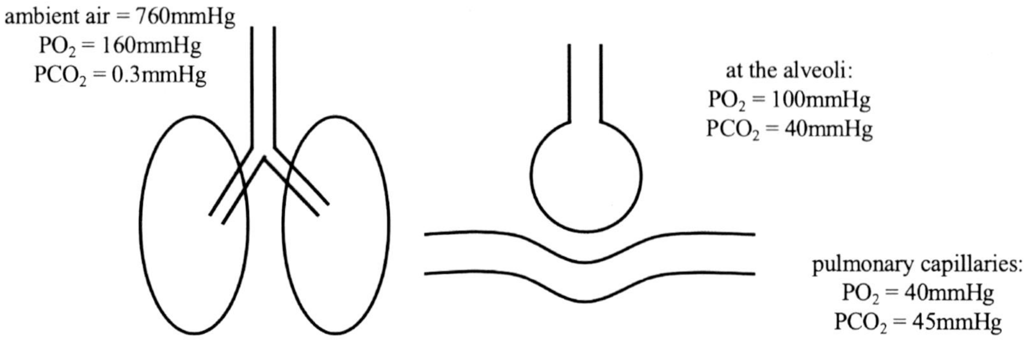

because there is an open system between the ambient air and the alveoli, the overall pressure at the alveoli is also 760mmHg at baseline, however the partial pressures of the components are different along the way

The pressure gradient or difference from alveolus to capillary is drastically different when comparing the two gasses: oxygen has a pressure difference of about 60mmHg, carbon dioxide has one of just 5mmHg. While this may seem, at first glance, to put the body at risk of some sort of imbalance, carbon dioxide moves more easily through the liquid membrane (roughly twenty times so) and the net result is that oxygen and carbon dioxide exchange at about the same rate.

[5] Betts & friends, 2013 – This chapter discusses these numbers in the context of Dalton's Law and lists all the values we used except for PO_2 at the alveoli; that one is cited as 104mmHg in their text, but we calculated it out in the **Appendix** and use our calculated value to maintain consistency throughout this text

[6] Speller, 2018 – Outlines how both oxygen and carbon dioxide diffuse in the pulmonary system within the context of gas laws; do note, however, that certain states can slow this process down (and we'll get to those later on)

PEEP – positive end-expiratory pressure; **PPV** – positive-pressure ventilation; **PCO_2** – partial pressure of carbon dioxide; **PO_2** – partial pressure of oxygen

How is Positive-Pressure Ventilation Different?

Now we need to consider what happens when we bypass the whole negative-pressure mechanism for ventilation and instead opt for a positive-pressure approach.[7] Let's start at the top with the basic sketch of airways and lungs superimposed on the chest wall and diaphragm. When we ventilate by positive-pressure ventilation (PPV) we have to physically displace the diaphragm and chest wall while simultaneously pushing air into the system. This requires a lot more pressure than we needed for that negative-pressure, spontaneous mechanism:

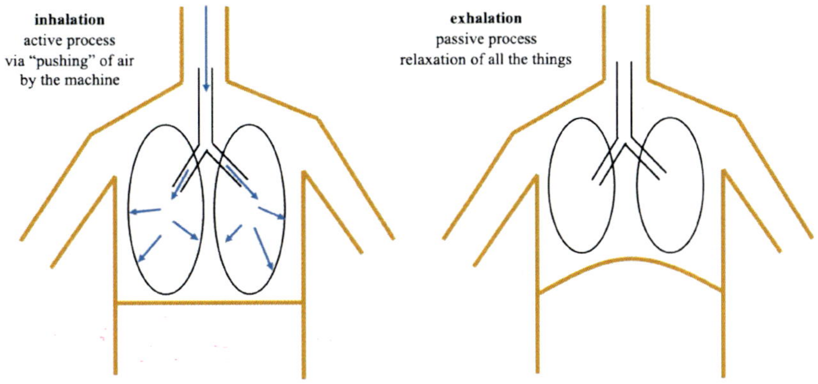

We will get to airway pressures and limits for them later on, but a normal **Plateau Pressure** (which reflects the average alveolar pressure in positive-pressure ventilation) is in the range of 15-25cm$H_2$0; compare this to the pressures represented in the following illustration:[8]

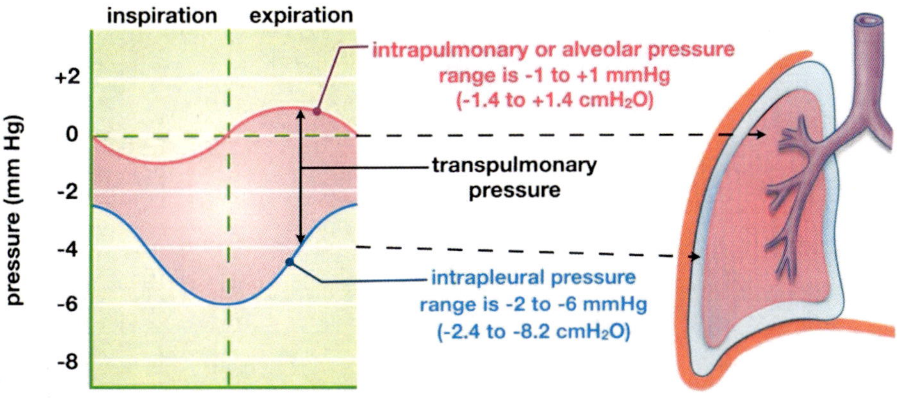

[7] This assumes that the patient is not contributing to this effort of breathing; to say it another way, this description is accurate for the patient who is not making any respiratory effort or is out of synch with mechanical efforts; in reality we can synch patient effort to machine effort to minimize the differences and effects discussed in this section (more on this in **Comfort**)

[8] We'll talk about the mmHg and cmH_2O conundrum at the end of the next section (in **Measuring Pressures**); alveolar pressure is the most relevant to our discussion for now, the concepts of transpulmonary pressure and intrapleural pressures are deferred here; graphic built by Dr. Sameer of *Art by Dr. Sam* on Fiverr and *The Young Orthopod* on YouTube

ARDS – acute respiratory distress syndrome; **cmH_2O** – centimeters of water; **CO_2** – carbon dioxide; **mmHg** – millimeters of mercury
O_2 – oxygen; **OK** – alright

The biggest impact of that increased intrathoracic pressure is the effect it can have on cardiac output. Increased intrathoracic pressure can decrease blood return to the heart via pressure on the vena cava, resulting in decreased preload and, therefore, less output.[9] Let's represent it this way:

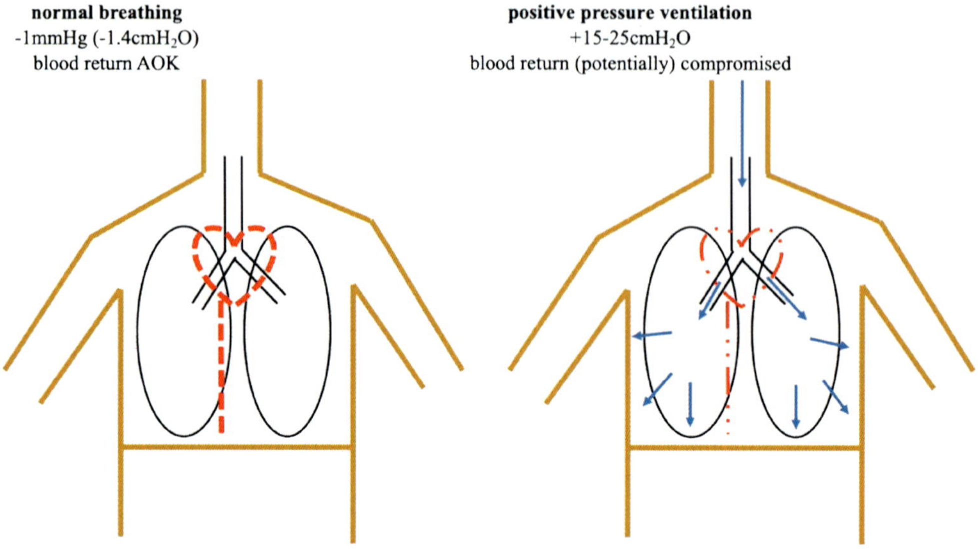

Other negative sequalae of positive-pressure ventilation (which may still occur even if we have all the settings dialed in right!) would be patient discomfort, muscle fatigue and/ or weakening,[10] and physiologic changes to other body systems.[11] And then if we have things dialed in wrong on the machine or don't ventilate appropriately based on patient presentation, we can also cause things like direct injury to the alveoli and hypoventilation (leading to shock). This is but a short list of the major things we'll worry about in this manual, just recognize that there is a lot of potential for bad and that's why we need to know how to manage the machine to the best of our collective ability and to mitigate as many of these things as we can along the way.

[9]Strong, 2013; Mahmood & Pinsky, 2018 – Both this video and the article explain in more detail on how positive-pressure ventilation (and particularly **Positive End-Expiratory Pressure**, discussed later) can affect cardiac output, especially with concurrent hypovolemia; while it isn't always true that positive pressure decreases cardiac output (sometimes the opposite can occur), the positive-pressure ventilation/ PEEP → decreased preload → decreased cardiac output sequence of events is most relevant to us in the transport setting

[10] Tobin & friends, 2010 – Outlines the idea that we can mitigate fatigue and weakening by adjusting vent settings to require that the patient make some intrinsic effort to breathe; while their ending advice is to utilize an airway pressure waveform to monitor patient effort (something we don't routinely have in the transport setting), it still provides valuable insight on the whole concept

[11] Yartsev, 2019 – In fact, navigate to the *Respiratory System* header at the top of this page and then down to the section on *Physiology of Positive Pressure Ventilation* for more detail on all of this stuff

PEEP – positive end-expiratory pressure; **PPV** – positive-pressure ventilation; **PCO_2** – partial pressure of carbon dioxide; **PO_2** – partial pressure of oxygen

We already saw how a pressure waveform might look over time with spontaneous, negative-pressure breaths, so let's see how it looks with a machine-delivered breath. Note that there are different types of machine-delivered breaths in this diagram (plus some terms to discuss), and we haven't yet gotten there; that's totally OK and we just want to point out some general trends here. Big takeaway: the left set of patterns (the normal) looks nice and smooth, without any harsh changes or drastic swings in amplitude; all of the others have those things we don't want. Another noteworthy point is that the graphic representations of the types of breaths (i.e. each column of the three towards the right) are each slightly different. Sometimes one mode or type of breath will be more comfortable for a certain patient in spite of trying to do all the other things we know how to do, simply because how that patient's body responds:[12]

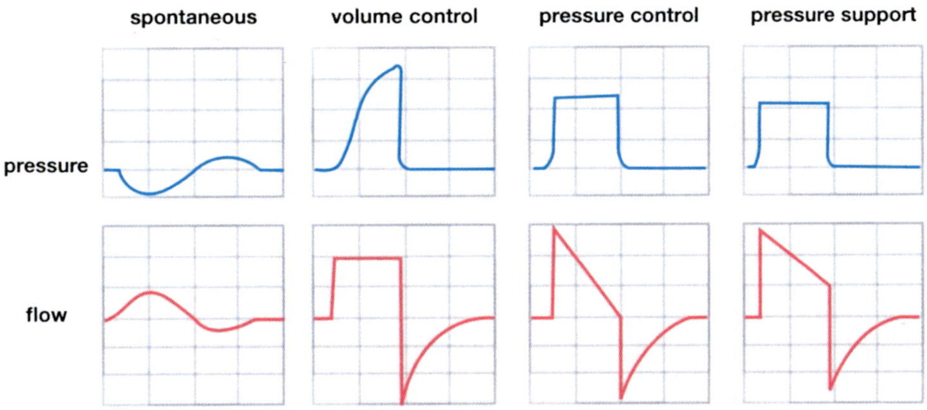

In an effort not to discourage anyone from ever putting a patient on a vent, there are advantages to positive-pressure ventilation and mechanical ventilation. Most obvious of these is that it allows us to breathe for a patient in a relatively simple way when that patient is unable to do so on his or her own. More specifically, mechanical ventilation allows us to control and direct recovery with specific conditions and diseases (such as acidosis, asthma, and ARDS – all of which we will discuss later on). Positive pressure can help move oxygen into the bloodstream more easily, managing ventilation can help that oxygen get delivered more effectively, manipulating time spent at different parts of the respiratory cycle can increase the amount of time that the body can participate in pulmonary respiration, etc. There are lots of good uses of the ventilator and we will get to all of them in due time, so don't worry if that got to be too much for a moment and know that in spite of its drawbacks, mechanical ventilation and does have its place in the cosmos.[13]

---

[12] This assessment of what the body wants in terms of smooth waveforms and avoidance of harsh changes in amplitude is a subjective concept - it seems to make intuitive sense, but there may not be a good way to verify the idea; graphic built by Dr. Sameer of *Art by Dr. Sam* on Fiverr and *The Young Orthopod* on YouTube

[13] Hill, 2019 – And if you need convincing that mechanical ventilation is preferred to simply using a bag-valve device, take a look at this discussion of a recent paper

ARDS – acute respiratory distress syndrome; **ATM** – atmosphere; **cm** – centimeter; **cmH₂O** – centimeters of water; **CO_2** – carbon dioxide; **COPD** – chronic obstructive pulmonary disease; **$EtCO_2$** – end-tidal carbon dioxide

Other Important Concepts

Terms to Describe Breathing

Just to differentiate the words that collectively describe breathing, let's chat about a few terms.[14] **Ventilation** refers to the gross movement of air as the body breathes in and out. **Oxygenation** refers to the transition of oxygen from the air outside of the body, through the respiratory and circulatory systems, and to the capillaries where it can be picked up by the tissues for use. Lastly is respiration, which has two specific types. Pulmonary respiration refers to the exchange of carbon dioxide and oxygen in the alveoli of the lungs; cellular respiration refers to a comparable gas exchange at the tissues. To visualize it all, here are a few images:

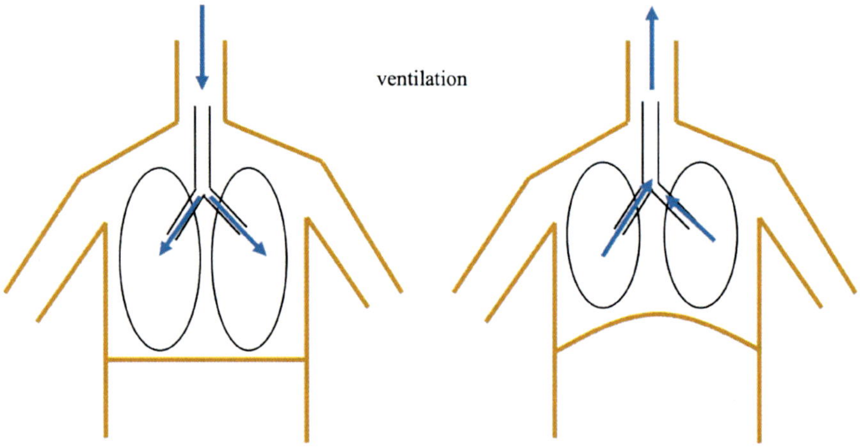

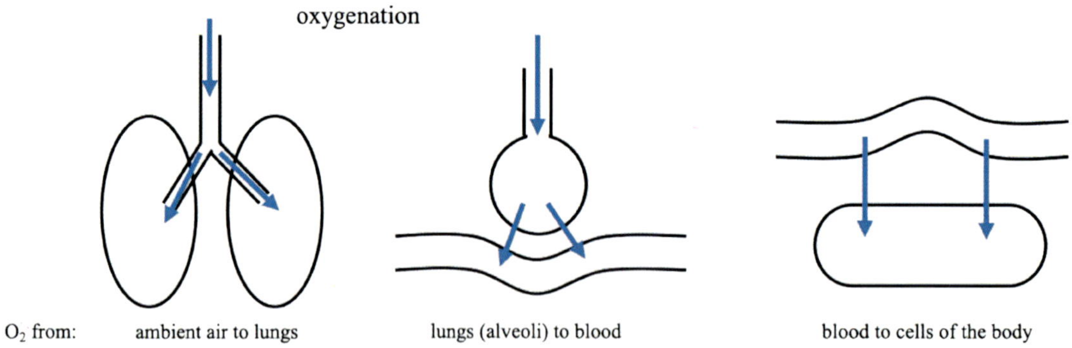

[14] Betts & friends, 2013 – Explains in more detail the processes of ventilation (Section 22.3) and respiration (Section 22.4)

IBW – ideal body weight; **kPa** – kilopascal; **kg** – kilograms; **lbs** – pounds; **ml** – milliliter; **mmHg** – millimeters of mercury; **O_2** – oxygen; **PBW** – predicted body weight; **PSI** – pounds per square inch

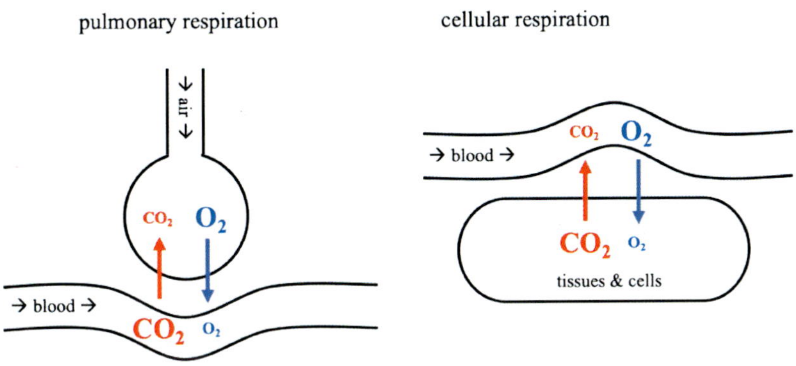

There is some overlap between oxygenation and pulmonary respiration in all of this, but it helps to separate these ideas. When managing the vent, we typically focus on the processes of ventilation and oxygenation. While respiration (in both forms) is very important, our ability to manipulate it isn't as straightforward as it is with ventilation and oxygenation. That said, we can actually influence all of these processes with the ventilator and we will point these things out as we get to them.[15]

[15] Hasudungan, 2018 – This video is a general recap of respiratory system physiology and the oxygen-hemoglobin dissociation curve, it sheds some insight on this idea that ventilation is intricately linked to both pulmonary and cellular respiration; we will reference it again when we discuss **Oxygenation**

ARDS – acute respiratory distress syndrome; **ATM** – atmosphere; **cm** – centimeter; **cmH$_2$O** – centimeters of water; **CO$_2$** – carbon dioxide; **COPD** – chronic obstructive pulmonary disease; **EtCO$_2$** – end-tidal carbon dioxide

Dead Space

Dead space can be an intimidating concept in vent management and we are going to try to both simplify it and identify specific situations in which it matters. To start with, there are four types of dead space that we will discuss: anatomic, alveolar, physiologic, and mechanical.[16] Dead space, as a term, can be used to describe any one of these subtypes, but it helps to recognize which type of dead space is of concern in a given situation. And know that we sometimes see dead space notated as V_D.

First of all, anatomic dead space is the air involved in the respiratory cycle that cannot participate in gas exchange. As represented by the blue lines, it starts at the naso- and oro-pharynxes and extends down to the terminal bronchioles:

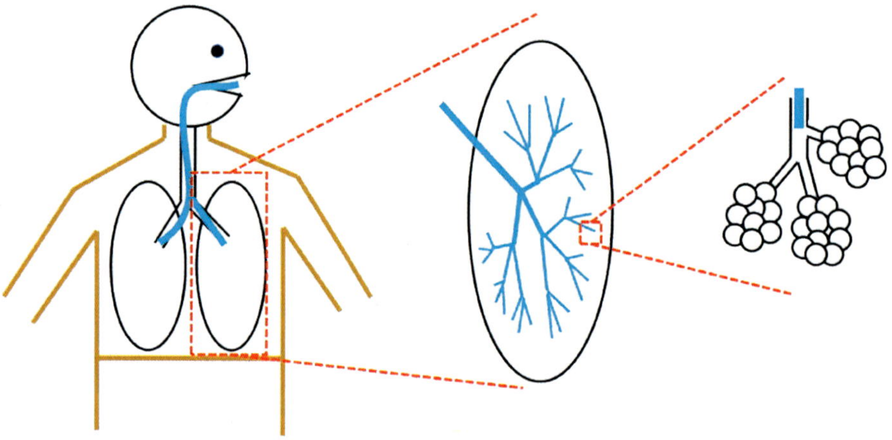

Another way to describe anatomic dead space, in light of this graphic, would be just about all the air involved in a breath other than what ends up in the alveoli and respiratory bronchioles. Now this graphic isn't to scale, so it sort of seems as if dead space is the majority of the air involved, but that isn't the case. There are over a thousand terminal bronchioles in a single lung and hundreds of millions of alveoli total, so the majority of air ends up in the alveoli.[17] It's also worth noting that this process is dynamic and that anatomic dead space refers to the air outside of the alveoli and respiratory bronchioles when those alveoli are fully inflated at peak inspiration.

---

[16] Yartsev, 2019 – This is the best content we've been able to find on this subject of dead space, very thorough and with references to more information along the way

[17] Betts & friends, 2013; Ochs & friends, 2003 – And just to clarify: the terminal bronchioles (marked by the thick blue line in the far right side of this graphic) are different than the respiratory bronchioles, which are the stems distal to that blue line that feed into each cluster of alveoli

IBW – ideal body weight; **kPa** – kilopascal; **kg** – kilograms; **lbs** – pounds; **ml** – milliliter; **mmHg** – millimeters of mercury; O_2 – oxygen; **PBW** – predicted body weight; **PSI** – pounds per square inch

Anatomic dead space is most relevant in our discussion of ventilated patients when we need to alter the amount of air that participates in alveolar gas exchange (i.e. **Ventilation**). We will talk about this more later, but we basically have two options when it comes to increasing this amount of air: increasing the frequency at which we deliver breaths or increasing the amount of air per breath delivered. If we add one breath to the equation, we must consider anatomic dead space and therefore the amount of air to the alveoli is less than the actual volume of that entire breath. On the other hand, if we simply add volume to breaths already being delivered, we get more of that additional volume at the alveoli because anatomic dead space has already been considered for each breath.[18]

The next type of dead space is alveolar dead space. Alveolar dead space refers to the air in the alveoli without a corresponding blood supply.[19] The classic example is an emboli that restricts blood flow to a portion of the lung. Other causes would include decreased cardiac output (i.e. shock) and chronic lung disease (i.e. COPD). It is worth mentioning that alveolar dead space is often described as an absolute thing, as in zero perfusion to a particular alveolus. In reality, however, there is a spectrum on which ventilation and perfusion can correlate. The details on that and a quantitative definition don't matter much in this discussion, but it is good to know that there is some variation in defining alveolar dead space.

In the normal human body, alveolar dead space is close to zero and we consider it to be negligible. For the sick or injured, however, we assume some alveolar dead space and proactively take steps to accommodate that. These actions, all of which we will touch on as we move forward, include ensuring adequate oxygenation,[20] judiciously applying end-expiratory pressure,[21] positioning the patient properly, and maintaining hemodynamic function to avoid shock states.[22] All of these things collectively maximize the efficacy of the ventilator treatment we are administering. In the event that no alveolar dead space existed before these interventions, no harm is done. All of these things are of benefit even in the absence of alveolar dead space, but they are particularly beneficial for those patients who do have some degree of it.

Next on the list is physiologic dead space. Physiologic dead space is the sum of anatomic dead space and alveolar dead space and represents all of the dead space before we introduce our devices into the system. In the healthy person, we often assume no alveolar dead space and therefore physiologic dead space is equal to anatomic dead space. The utility of knowing physiologic dead space is that it can be measured and then used to calculate or estimate those other two kinds of dead space: alveolar and anatomic.[23] But given that this isn't normally a possibility in transport, the utility of describing dead space this way doesn't much help our treatment. That said, from here on out we will refer to anatomic dead space and alveolar dead space in an effort to be more specific with our discussion.

---

[18] There are some nuances to this idea of how dead space varies with volume delivered, but we'll cover those later on in **Volume Control**, **Tidal Volume**, and the **Appendix**

[19] Mason, 2019 – For an alternative explanation of alveolar dead space, refer to this short video

[20] This idea of mitigating dead space via **Oxygenation** ties into the very next section on **Hypoxic Pulmonary Vasoconstriction**

[21] Murias & friends, 2014 – As outlined in this article, **Positive End-Expiratory Pressure** can reduce alveolar dead space, but only to a certain point; after that, further increases will create more of it

[22] Yartsev, 2019 – Among many other things, this article describes how we can reduce alveolar dead space by both positioning the patient appropriately and maintaining perfusion

[23] Johnston, 2015 – This article reviews techniques by which we can measure physiologic dead space and then use it to determine a value for anatomic dead space

Last type of dead space is what we will call mechanical dead space. Mechanical dead space, which may also be noted as equipment or apparatus dead space, is the dead space that we add on to the system with our devices: vent circuit, end-tidal carbon dioxide ($EtCO_2$) detector, heat & moister exchanger (HME) or humidifier, etc.[24] To be a bit more specific, it refers to all the things from where anatomic dead space starts (oropharynx/ nasopharynx) to where exhaled air leaves the wye of the vent circuit:

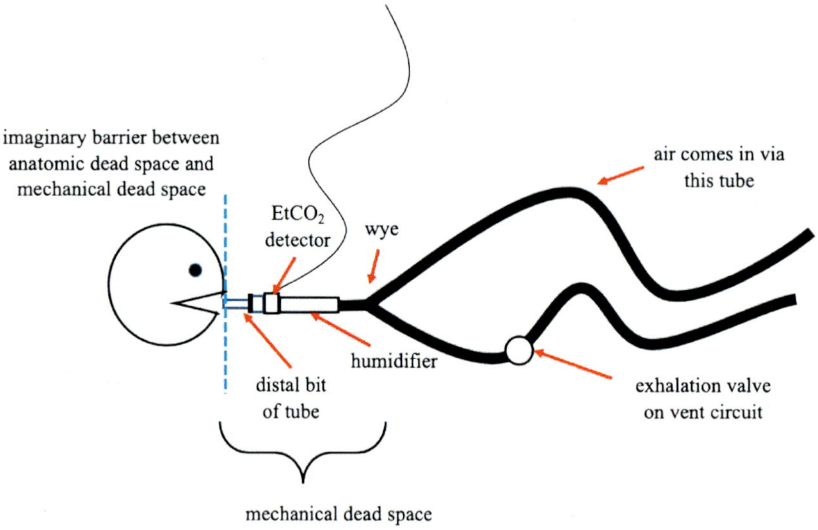

Mechanical dead space is a problem because it increases the amount of used-up air with which incoming air must be mixed before it gets to the alveoli. In the normal human being, fresh air is pulled into the airways starting right at that imaginary blue line in the above picture; in the ventilated patient, fresh air begins at that wye. We've discussed this effect in the **Appendix**, but suffice it to say that we should try to minimize mechanical dead space when possible (i.e. think about whether or not an in-line suction device or humidifier is needed rather than placing them blindly for all patients) and that the effect is more pronounced with smaller patients and higher respiratory rates (i.e. pediatrics).

One last thing about this is that there is a silver lining to our concept of mechanical dead space. The endotracheal tube actually creates a narrow passageway from the teeth/ lips (where we drew that blue line) down to the trachea, essentially negating the dead space of the naso- and oro-pharynxes. So while the net change in overall dead space may be negligible as far as amount added versus amount taken away, we still want to maximize efficacy of ventilation and minimize unnecessary things in our vent circuit when possible.

There is another related concept to consider in this discussion of dead space that doesn't quite fit any of the types mentioned above. We like to think of all of these volumes as fixed quantities of air, but the truth is that the containers that hold this air are flexible or have stretch and therefore we sometimes see differences in expected versus actual values. One example of this is that the amount of air we put into the system doesn't always match up exactly with air out of the system.[25] So where does that air go? Some of it stays in the alveoli (see upcoming discussion on recruitment), some of it leaks around our cuff, some of it is lost to the tissues and airway structures, etc. While this isn't exactly dead space per se, it helps to recognize that it is a thing that can cloud our understanding of air volumes.

---

[24] Heat & moisture exchangers will be discussed in detail when we get to **Humidifiers**

[25] This difference between tidal volume and exhaled tidal volume will be addressed in **Volume Control** and then expanded on in **Tidal Volume**

IBW – ideal body weight; **kPa** – kilopascal; **kg** – kilograms; **lbs** – pounds; **ml** – milliliter; **mmHg** – millimeters of mercury; O_2 – oxygen; **PBW** – predicted body weight; **PSI** – pounds per square inch

Another place where this comes into play is with the vent circuits themselves. These plastic tubes are not rigid and do have a certain amount of stretch to them. If we look at the package of the tubing, there is a value that says how much volume of stretch a given circuit has per unit of pressure. We will revisit this idea in later sections once we discuss a few of the concepts mentioned here, but know that in certain types of ventilation we may inadvertently overestimate the amount of air delivered if we ignore the stretch of the circuit. This is particularly relevant with little patients (i.e. infants), as the impact of this effect (ratio of misestimation to potential outcome) is more pronounced with smaller breaths.[26]

Hypoxic Pulmonary Vasoconstriction[27]

Hypoxia results in vasoconstriction of the pulmonary vascular bed (thus the term hypoxic pulmonary vasoconstriction), which is opposite of what happens in systemic circulation. This mechanism helps the lungs avoid wasting blood supply to part of the lung that isn't getting enough oxygen – it's a mechanism to conserve resources and maximize efficiency in the system. Just as with other vascular beds in the body, the pulmonary capillaries are in a constant state of flux and respond to the needs of the body and the availability of resources (oxygen, in this case, being the driving force) by opening and closing.

Carrying on this conversation with a new term: hypoxic pulmonary vasoconstriction helps to avoid ventilation/ perfusion (V/Q) mismatch, which could look like either of the following:[28]

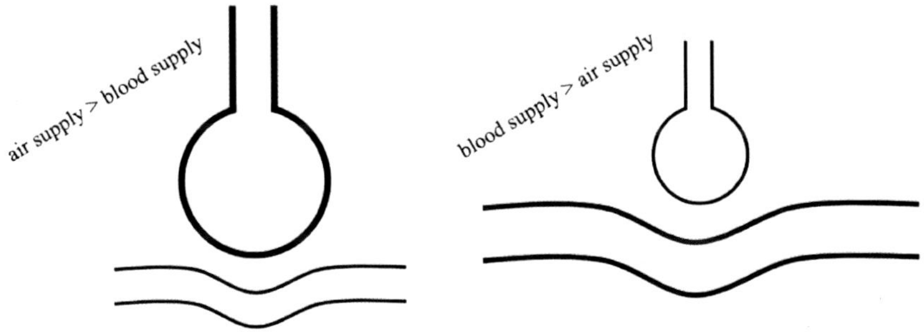

[26] Bauer, 2018 – He discusses this idea of stretch in the vent circuit in his book on vent management; we also mention it in our discussion of **Volume Control** and then demonstrate this impact in the context of managing a pediatric patient later on in the **Appendix**

[27] For more reading on the subject of hypoxic pulmonary vasoconstriction:
Dunham-Snary & friends, 2017 – They describe how this response can be inhibited by certain interventions and discuss the role of hypoxic pulmonary vasoconstriction in different pathologies
Lumb & Slinger, 2015 – This paper outlines the timelines discussed and also points out a number of relevant pharmacologic agents that contribute to the effect

[28] Mason, 2019 - We just left out the idea of ventilation/ perfusion (V/Q) ratio in this discussion because our focus is on the general idea only, but take a look here for a quick explanation

ARDS – acute respiratory distress syndrome; **ATM** – atmosphere; **cm** – centimeter; **cmH$_2$O** – centimeters of water; **CO$_2$** – carbon dioxide; **COPD** – chronic obstructive pulmonary disease; **EtCO$_2$** – end-tidal carbon dioxide

The left side type of ventilation/ perfusion (V/Q) mismatch demonstrates alveolar dead space. It shows that air supply (i.e. oxygen) in the alveolus is in excess of blood flow and therefore some of that oxygen won't get utilized or move into the bloodstream. The right side state is what we call a shunt. In a shunt, blood ends up passing through the pulmonary vascular bed without getting its full complement of oxygen. It isn't always the case that the mismatch is due to volume of air in the alveoli as shown, it can also be related to some kind of impediment that prevents the movement of air out of the alveoli. Examples of this would be pulmonary edema, ARDS, and pneumonia. In either of these cases, dead space or shunt, hypoxic pulmonary vasoconstriction is one of the body's mechanisms for either reversing or avoiding these types of mismatches.

Now one thing to know about this whole process is that it goes both ways: vasoconstriction is the response to hypoxia and vasodilation occurs when oxygenation is adequate or that hypoxic state is resolved. We might consider these to be similar processes, just in opposite directions. There is a distinction, however, in the rate at which either change happens. The initial hypoxic vasoconstriction side of things happens on the order of second to minutes; the reverse process (vasodilation) typically also occurs quickly, but can happen much more slowly (up to hours) or incompletely (without complete reversal of the vasoconstriction) when the hypoxic pulmonary vasoconstriction response has been sustained for a while.

The fact that it may take quite some time to reverse this process helps to explain, in part, why we aren't always able to fix our vented patients as well as we want to in the short span we get to hang with them in transport. It also helps bring out the idea that just because a patient doesn't look awesome when we get there doesn't mean that the sending facility or crew has been doing things wrong – they may be taking the right steps and called us before enough time passed for the fix to work its way out. There are many more intricacies and effects of hypoxic pulmonary vasoconstriction on the body (see all those references on the previous page), but the main point is that we may not be able to fix a super sick patient quickly. And that's just fine. We do what we can (as we will outline soon) and recognize that there are limits to the results we can expect.

IBW – ideal body weight; **kPa** – kilopascal; **kg** – kilograms; **lbs** – pounds; **ml** – milliliter; **mmHg** – millimeters of mercury; O_2 – oxygen; **PBW** – predicted body weight; **PSI** – pounds per square inch

Alveolar Surface Area

Even though we have been demonstrating the alveoli-capillary interface as a single blood vessel running past an air sac, it is important to recognize, again, that this is a simplification of how things are and that the surface of the alveoli are covered by a network of vessels:[29]

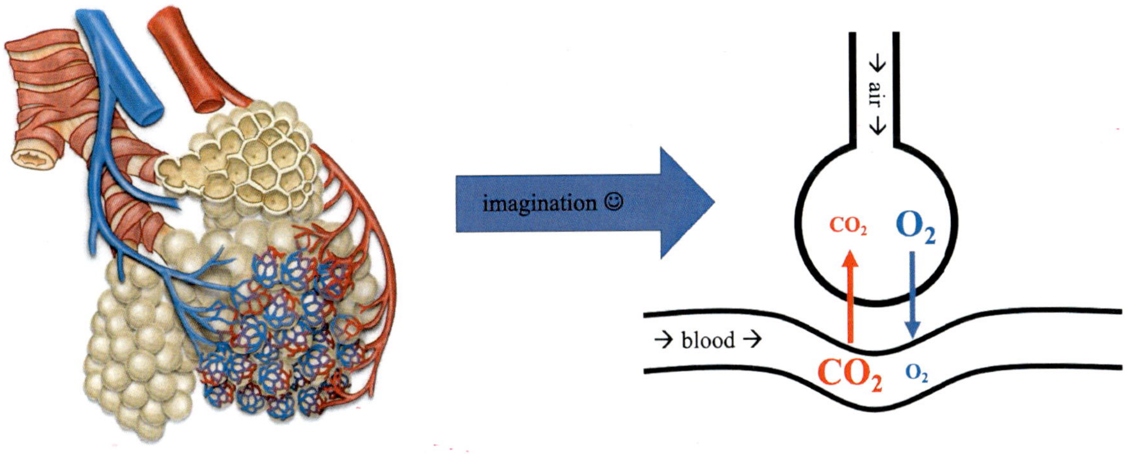

When we inflate the alveoli we get more surface area and that means more interface between air and blood. In addition, inflation of the alveoli causes the alveolar membrane to stretch and become thinner, allowing for easier diffusion of gasses:[30]

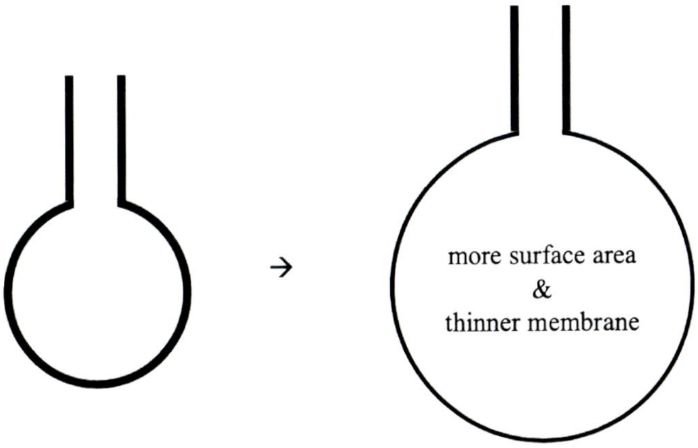

[29] Left bit of this graphic built by Dr. Sameer of *Art by Dr. Sam* on Fiverr and *The Young Orthopod* on YouTube

[30] Desai, 2012 – We spell out this diffusion process in much more detail in the section on **Oxygenation**, but here's a video to explain how these factors are related to gas exchange across the alveolar-capillary membrane

ARDS – acute respiratory distress syndrome; **ATM** – atmosphere; **cm** – centimeter; **cmH_2O** – centimeters of water; **CO_2** – carbon dioxide; **COPD** – chronic obstructive pulmonary disease; **EtCO_2** – end-tidal carbon dioxide

More surface area and a thinner membrane make it easier to move air from inside of the alveoli to the circulatory system, so lots of our interventions with the vent are focused on this idea. That said, certain things can get in the way of this gas exchange even if we do get the surface area up and membrane thinned out. Think of these as things that impact access to usable alveolar surface area:[31]

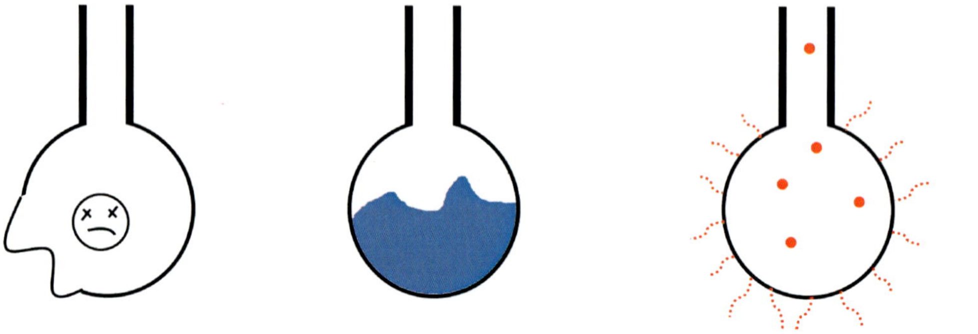

toxins can injure the membrane directly | fluid can impede gas exchange across the membrane | inflammation can damage the membrane and impair diffusion

Now are there are ways to work through these impediments and we'll talk about strategies to make that happen later.[32] Also know that while more alveolar surface is important, if taken too far it we can cause over-inflation injury or barotrauma that results in damage to this membrane. How we maintain safety of the alveoli is something we'll get to later on.[33] For now we'll summarize it like this: management of the alveolar surface is important for gas exchange and there are both interventions we can take to improve the efficiency of gas diffusion across that membrane and steps to take to maintain safety and avoid causing further damage.

---

[31] George, 2015 – Check this out for a bit of extra detail on the difference between pneumonia and pneumonitis, both of which would be included in this working list of things that can inhibit effective gas exchange

[32] Strategies to facilitate gas exchange are discussed in the section on **Oxygenation**

[33] We talk about ensuring alveolar safety in many places in this manual, but mostly in the sections on **Control of Ventilation** and **Plateau Pressure**

IBW – ideal body weight; **kPa** – kilopascal; **kg** – kilograms; **lbs** – pounds; **ml** – milliliter; **mmHg** – millimeters of mercury; **O_2** – oxygen; **PBW** – predicted body weight; **PSI** – pounds per square inch

Ideal Body Weight

Second to last thing before we move on to talking about the machine: lung size is most strongly correlated with patient height. Because of this, we use a patient's height to calculate an ideal body weight (IBW) when doing vent things.[34] The idea is that a six-foot human could weigh either 120lbs or 300lbs and the size of his or her lungs wouldn't change. There is a formula to calculate IBW for both males and females, often presented as a hybrid of metric and standard units:

$$IBW_{male}\ (kg) = (2.3(\text{height in inches}) - 60) + 50$$
$$IBW_{female}\ (kg) = (2.3(\text{height in inches}) - 60) + 45.5$$

For the metric enthusiasts, we also have it as so:

$$IBW_{male}\ (kg) = (0.91(\text{height in cm}) - 152.4) + 50$$
$$IBW_{female}\ (kg) = (0.91(\text{height in cm}) - 152.4) + 45.5$$

Or we can use charts like this:[35]

HEIGHT	PBW	4 ml	5 ml	6 ml	7 ml	8 ml
4' 0" (48)	17.9	72	90	107	125	143
4' 1" (49)	20.2	81	101	121	141	162
4' 2" (50)	22.5	90	113	135	158	180
4' 3" (51)	24.8	99	124	149	174	198
4' 4" (52)	27.1	108	136	163	190	217
4' 5" (53)	29.4	118	147	176	206	235
4' 6" (54)	31.7	127	159	190	222	254
4' 7" (55)	34	136	170	204	238	272
4' 8" (56)	36.3	145	182	218	254	290
4' 9" (57)	38.6	154	193	232	270	309
4' 10" (58)	40.9	164	205	245	286	327
4' 11" (59)	43.2	173	216	259	302	346
5' 0" (60)	45.5	182	228	273	319	364
5' 1" (61)	47.8	191	239	287	335	382
5' 2" (62)	50.1	200	251	301	351	401
5' 3" (63)	52.4	210	262	314	367	419
5' 4" (64)	54.7	219	274	328	383	438
5' 5" (65)	57	228	285	342	399	456
5' 6" (66)	59.3	237	297	356	415	474
5' 7" (67)	61.6	246	308	370	431	493
5' 8" (68)	63.9	256	320	383	447	511
5' 9" (69)	66.2	265	331	397	463	530
5' 10" (70)	68.5	274	343	411	480	548
5' 11" (71)	70.8	283	354	425	496	566
6' 0" (72)	73.1	292	366	439	512	585
6' 1" (73)	75.4	302	377	452	528	603
6' 2" (74)	77.7	311	389	466	544	622
6' 3" (75)	80	320	400	480	560	640
6' 4" (76)	82.3	329	412	494	576	658
6' 5" (77)	84.6	338	423	508	592	677
6' 6" (78)	86.9	348	435	521	608	695
6' 7" (79)	89.2	357	446	535	624	714
6' 8" (80)	91.5	366	458	549	641	732
6' 9" (81)	93.8	375	469	563	657	750
6' 10" (82)	96.1	384	481	577	673	769
6' 11" (83)	98.4	394	492	590	689	787
7' 0" (84)	100.7	403	504	604	705	806

PBW and Tidal Volume for Females

ARDSNet Studies

HEIGHT	PBW	4 ml	5 ml	6 ml	7 ml	8 ml
4' 0" (48)	22.4	90	112	134	157	179
4' 1" (49)	24.7	99	124	148	173	198
4' 2" (50)	27	108	135	162	189	216
4' 3" (51)	29.3	117	147	176	205	234
4' 4" (52)	31.6	126	158	190	221	253
4' 5" (53)	33.9	136	170	203	237	271
4' 6" (54)	36.2	145	181	217	253	290
4' 7" (55)	38.5	154	193	231	270	308
4' 8" (56)	40.8	163	204	245	286	326
4' 9" (57)	43.1	172	216	259	302	345
4' 10" (58)	45.4	182	227	272	318	363
4' 11" (59)	47.7	191	239	286	334	382
5' 0" (60)	50	200	250	300	350	400
5' 1" (61)	52.3	209	262	314	366	418
5' 2" (62)	54.6	218	273	328	382	437
5' 3" (63)	56.9	228	285	341	398	455
5' 4" (64)	59.2	237	296	355	414	474
5' 5" (65)	61.5	246	308	369	431	492
5' 6" (66)	63.8	255	319	383	447	510
5' 7" (67)	66.1	264	331	397	463	529
5' 8" (68)	68.4	274	342	410	479	547
5' 9" (69)	70.7	283	354	424	495	566
5' 10" (70)	73	292	365	438	511	584
5' 11" (71)	75.3	301	377	452	527	602
6' 0" (72)	77.6	310	388	466	543	621
6' 1" (73)	79.9	320	400	479	559	639
6' 2" (74)	82.2	329	411	493	575	658
6' 3" (75)	84.5	338	423	507	592	676
6' 4" (76)	86.8	347	434	521	608	694
6' 5" (77)	89.1	356	446	535	624	713
6' 6" (78)	91.4	366	457	548	640	731
6' 7" (79)	93.7	375	469	562	656	750
6' 8" (80)	96	384	480	576	672	768
6' 9" (81)	98.3	393	492	590	688	786
6' 10" (82)	100.6	402	503	604	704	805
6' 11" (83)	102.9	412	515	617	720	823
7' 0" (84)	105.2	421	526	631	736	842

PBW and Tidal Volume for Males

ARDSNet Studie

[34] IBW may also be referred to as predicted body weight (PBW)
[35] NHLBI ARDS Network, 2005 (image)

ARDS – acute respiratory distress syndrome; **ATM** – atmosphere; **cm** – centimeter; **cmH_2O** – centimeters of water; **CO_2** – carbon dioxide; **COPD** – chronic obstructive pulmonary disease; **$EtCO_2$** – end-tidal carbon dioxide

Some people remember this formula for ideal body weight as "inches over five feet" as shown below. The only problem with this is that it gets tricky if we have someone under five feet, but either way works:

$$IBW_{male}\ (kg) = 2.3(\text{every inch over } 5') + 50$$
$$IBW_{female}\ (kg) = 2.3(\text{every inch over } 5') + 45.5$$

When dealing with pediatric patients, our go-to reference is often the Broselow Tape, but we do have some formulas we can refer to if that isn't available:[36]

Infant Weight (kg) = 0.5(age in months) + 4
Little Kid (1 – 4 years) Weight (kg) = 2(age in years + 5)
Big Kid (5 – 14 years) Weight (kg) = 4(age in years)

And note that the Broselow overlaps with the equations and chart above, so if we have a small grownup or a big kid we should still be able to get an ideal body weight just fine. And very last thing: there are some apps out there that can help with this sort of thing, both for adults and for pediatrics.[37]

[36] Graves & friends, 2014 – There are lots of formulas out there to estimate weights for pediatrics, but we went with recommendations from these guys based on this paper they did comparing different methods

[37] Critical-Medical Guide & Pedi STAT – Both are excellent resources to have on hand for quickly referencing relevant things

IBW – ideal body weight; **kPa** – kilopascal; **kg** – kilograms; **lbs** – pounds; **ml** – milliliter; **mmHg** – millimeters of mercury; O_2 – oxygen; **PBW** – predicted body weight; **PSI** – pounds per square inch

Measuring Pressures

During mechanical ventilation we measure pressures in centimeters of water (cmH_2O). We may occasionally hear this pronounced as "sonnimeters" of water and know that a sonnimeter and a centimeter, in this context, are the same thing. So we have cmH_2O with mechanical ventilation, but we generally talk about ambient air pressures in other terms, such as mmHg, kPa, PSI, etc. We skimmed right on past this concept in a previous section when we said that 1mmHg is about $1.4cmH_20$,[38] but let's now put it all down in a chart just to make things clear:[39]

	ATM	PSI	kPa	mmHg	cmH_2O
ATM	1	14.7	101.3	760	1033
PSI	0.068	1	6.89	51.7	70.3
kPa	0.0099	0.145	1	7.5	10.2
mmHg	0.0013	0.019	0.133	1	1.36
cmH_2O	0.00097	0.014	0.098	0.736	1

Also, note that we assume ambient pressure as it relates to airway and vent stuff is zero; so while true atmospheric pressure at sea level is 760mmHg (1 ATM), we call it $0cmH_2O$ to make things easier.[40] And then we have a way to represent breaths we give as waveforms showing pressure as a function of time with this new zero point (representing atmospheric pressure) as the baseline. For now we are going to ignore **Positive End-Expiratory Pressure** (since we haven't discussed it yet); we also don't have to worry about the specific components of the waveform – all those things will be discussed later on:

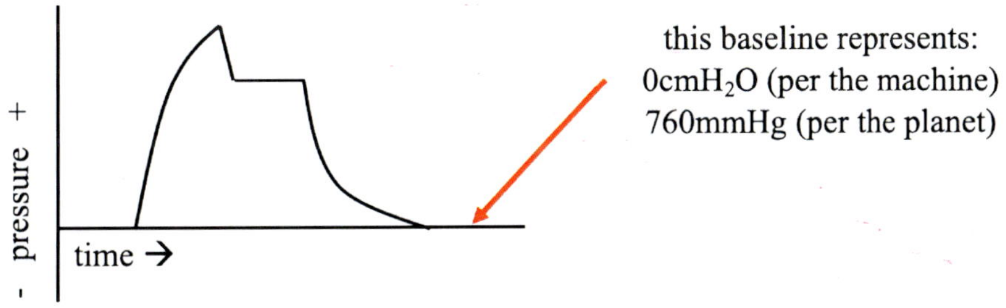

---

[38] This was in **How is Positive-Pressure Ventilation Different?** when we were talking about the fact that a negative-pressure, spontaneous breath only takes -1mmHg of pull while a typical positive-pressure breath via the machine takes $15\text{-}25cmH_20$ to move an equivalent amount of air

[39] We built this chart by Googling conversions for these values…

[40] Yartsev, 2019 – Scroll down to the section called *Airway Pressure* for some interesting background on why we measure and label pressures the way we do

Modes of Ventilation

This next section discusses how we organize the delivery of breaths to a patient. We've distinguished this concept of mode with that of control (see next section) in order to make things easier to conceptualize, but the terms sometimes get used with a bit of overlap. In reality, both the way we control breaths and how we organize those breaths are components of how we describe what mode we are in. While we could alternatively label this idea (what we refer to here as modes of ventilation) as breath sequence, the convention in transport is to identify this idea using the term mode, so we'll stick with that. Moving forward, we will refer to mode as the overall pattern or organization of breaths and control as the specific way we choose to deliver them.[41]

Before we get there, however, there is one concept that will be needed in order to understand things in the next few sections. **Triggers** are the thresholds by which the machine knows when to give a breath. We will talk about these in detail much later, but it is tough to explain the following ideas without a basic comprehension. In its simplest form, a trigger could simply be a quantity of time. An example of this would be one breath given every four seconds; we could then describe those instances as time-triggered breaths. There are also ways we can infer inspiratory effort made by the patient and have the machine give breaths based on those cues. We'll discuss how that happens later, but the general term for this type of thing is a patient trigger (i.e. a patient-triggered breath) and we will use that idea shortly.

[41] Chatburn & friends, 2014 – For specifics on how all of these modes and concepts of ventilation ought to be labeled and described, this article outlines a taxonomy for vent things

PS – pressure support; **SIMV** – synchronized intermittent mandatory ventilation

Basic Modes of Ventilation

The simplest way to ventilate a patient with a machine is to give breaths on a schedule and to ignore what the patient does on his or her own. Let's assume a hypothetical timeline running left to right over an arbitrary amount of time with black hashes to represent time-triggered breaths:

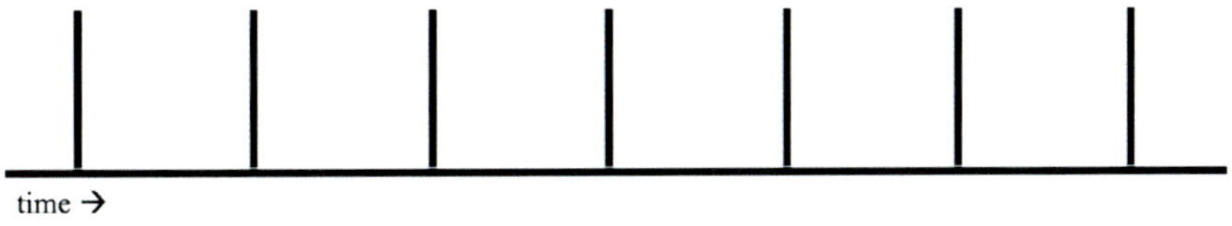

Now if the patient tries to take breaths overtop of this timeline, that effort gets ignored. We'll show it like this:

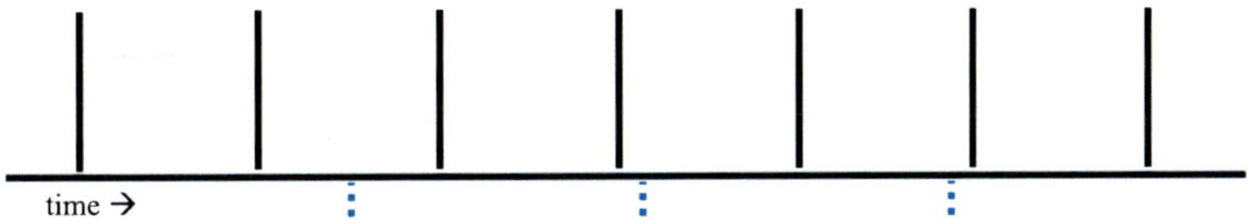

In terms of triggers, we could say that ventilation via this mechanism utilizes time triggers only and does not have a mechanism for patient triggers. Now there are two versions of this type of ventilation, controlled mechanical ventilation and intermittent mandatory ventilation (IMV).[42] The difference here is subtle: in controlled mechanical ventilation (which precedes all the other modes), the patient is physically unable to draw a breath on his or her own with effort made; in intermittent mandatory ventilation (a subsequent technological improvement) the patient is, in fact, able to draw a breath, it's just that the machine doesn't offer support and instead allows the patient to draw in air from the vent circuit independently and without help.

Controlled mechanical ventilation isn't routinely used, but it does get utilized in surgical settings when patients are paralyzed and for sure not making an effort to breathe spontaneously. Intermittent mandatory ventilation, on the other hand, is normally not available on its own – it typically comes with additional features which we will line out in just a bit. Now we may be able to manipulate our vent to approximate either of these modes in the event that we want to ignore patient triggers altogether, but those would be specific cases and we'll get to them later on.[43]

Moving on, subsequent modes build upon this framework by introducing mechanisms to support the patient's effort to breathe. When we introduce patient triggers, however, there is the potential that harm can result and we will talk about how different modes work to mitigate that risk. That said, utilizing the machine to augment patient effort improves comfort, facilitates recovery, reduces the negative effects of positive-pressure ventilation, and gives us more control over the management of the patient.[44] So now let's get on to the two modes commonly used in transport that take us beyond the basics and allow us to use patient triggers.

---

[42] Frakes, 2007; Kacmarek & Branson, 2016 – We won't refer to controlled mechanical ventilation as CMV (even though you sometimes see it that way), because CMV more often refers to continuous mandatory ventilation which we describe in just a moment; for more on this refer to both articles referenced

[43] These cases in which we might want to ignore patient-triggers are discussed in both **Overbreathing** and **Acute Deterioration**

[44] Mauri & friends, 2017; Goligher, 2017 – We will talk about the specific ways in which patient-triggered breaths are of benefit later on (in **Comfort**), but the article and essay provide a bit of context for these claims

AutoPEEP – intrinsic positive end-expiratory pressure; **OK** – alright

Assist Control

Assist control (AC), also known as continuous mandatory ventilation (CMV), is a mode that augments a patient's spontaneous respiratory effort by delivering a preset amount of air when an inspiratory effort is detected. To describe it in terms of triggers: time-triggered breaths are given on a schedule, but patient-triggered breaths can also occur in addition to those. Here's how it would look mapped out graphically:

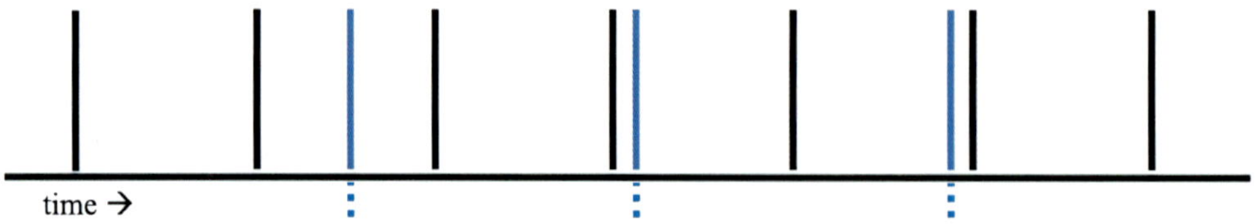

In assist control, all breaths are the same size. This means that patient-triggered breaths are the same (in terms of volume or pressure, see upcoming sections) as the machine-delivered, time-triggered ones. The obvious advantage here is that the patient's expressed need for more air per unit time is readily met. On the other hand, this method of giving full breaths whenever a trigger is sense has the potential to cause some harm. To start to make sense of this, let's return back to a series of time-triggered breaths with effort notated by dotted lines below the timeline. In assist control each instance of patient effort (whether true patient effort or simply perceived patient effort due to some other factor) has a varying potential for harm based on where it lines up in relation to other breaths. We'll draw it out first and then explain in detail:

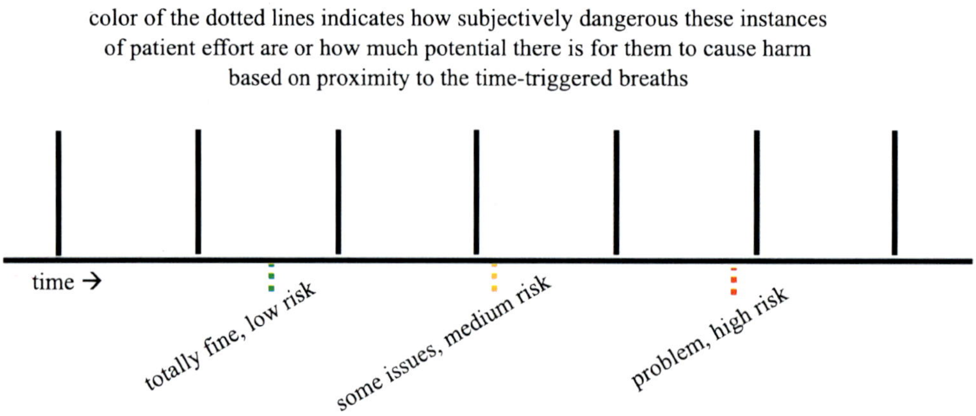

PS – pressure support; **SIMV** – synchronized intermittent mandatory ventilation

To expand on this: with the green effort, there is space (in time) on either side of the breath, so the machine can actualize that breath without affecting other breaths in proximity:

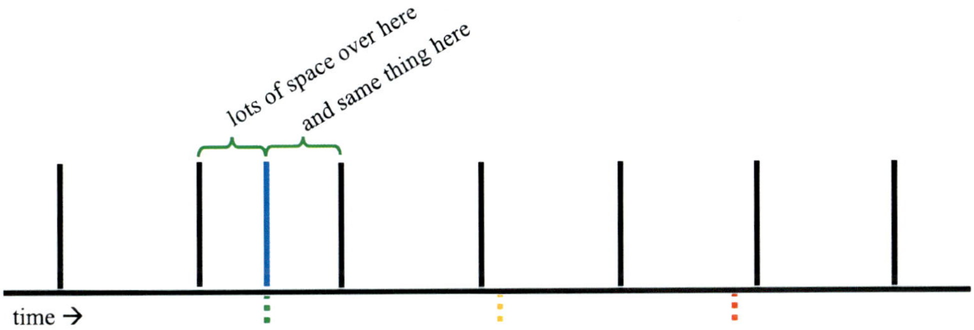

The difference between that green, patient-triggered breath and the baseline, time-triggered ones can be represented via those pressure-over-time waveforms that we mentioned before. Note the dip at the start of the second waveform as the patient breathes in – this is the effort that gets sensed by the machine right before a full positive-pressure breath is then given:[45]

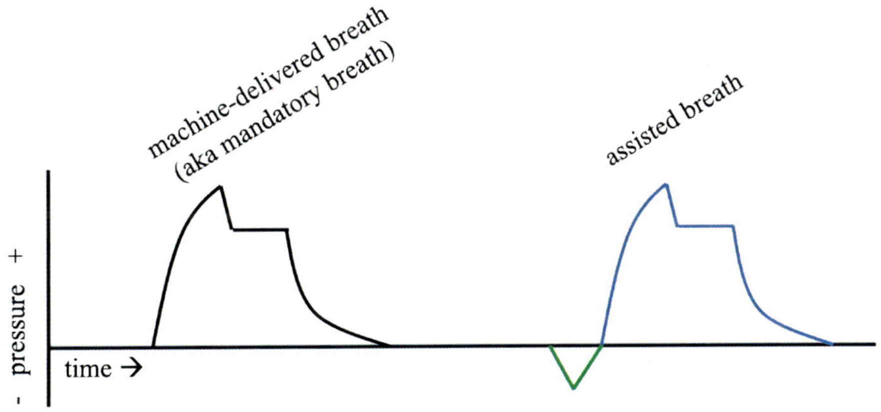

A pretty good assist control situation might look something like this where the patient's need for more breaths is generally met and that need, in the form of inspiratory effort, doesn't interfere or overlap with the scheduled breaths:

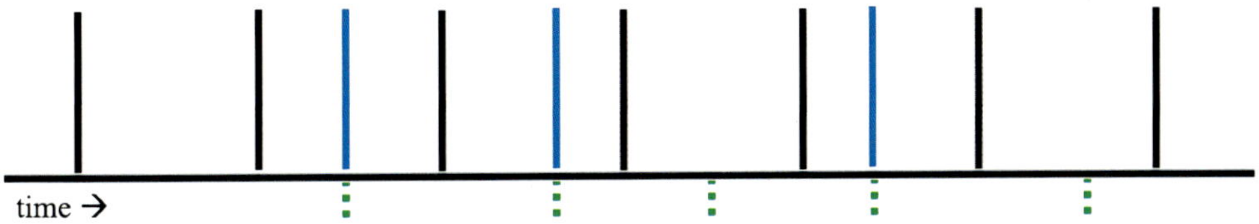

[45] Now this graphic makes it seem as if a pressure change detected by the machine leads to an assisted breath; while that could potentially be the case, the more common situation is a flow trigger (see **Triggers** for more)

AutoPEEP – intrinsic positive end-expiratory pressure; **OK** – alright

Do note that not all patient effort will result in delivered breaths. That's where triggers come in and we can adjust that parameter to make it more or less likely that a breath will occur. Again, more on this later, just something to note for now. And the ideal assist control situation (in contrast to the pretty good one shown above) would be when all patient effort results in a delivered breath, none of those patient-triggered breaths interfere with the time-triggered ones, and when no miscellaneous factors cause accidental triggers. No need to draw that one out, as it will be much clearer later on. For now we want to stay on track with describing assist control and how we can potentially cause harm in this mode.

In the case of the yellow effort (which we labeled as medium risk) there is a potential trigger that immediately follows another breath. It could be that the other breath in question is a machine-delivered one (as we had it in the first graphic) or it could be another patient-triggered one:

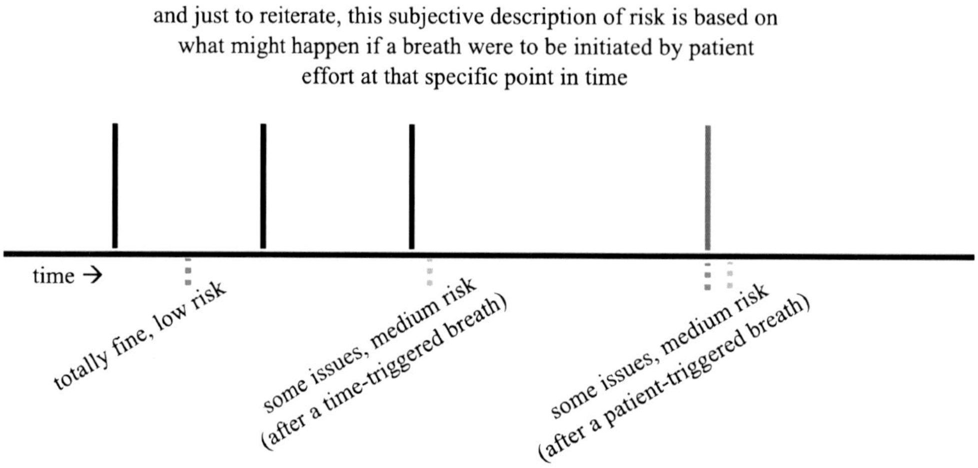

Now what happens next depends largely on how the trigger is set up, but we can generalize it by saying that the further along the first breath is or the closer the breath is to an end-exhalation baseline, the more likely that the effort will catch and result in a full breath. There are two possible outcomes: one in which the trigger results in an assisted breath and one in which the trigger does not result in a breath:[46]

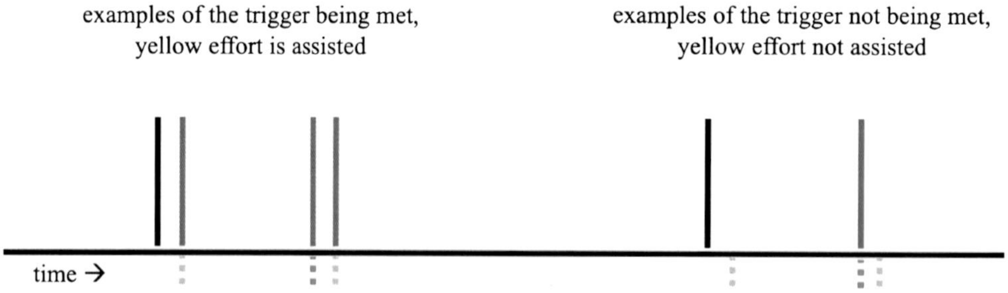

[46] And as already mentioned, we will discuss this idea of **Triggers** in much more detail later

PS – pressure support; **SIMV** – synchronized intermittent mandatory ventilation

And then we can carry on with the idea to show either of those outcomes as a waveform of pressure over time:

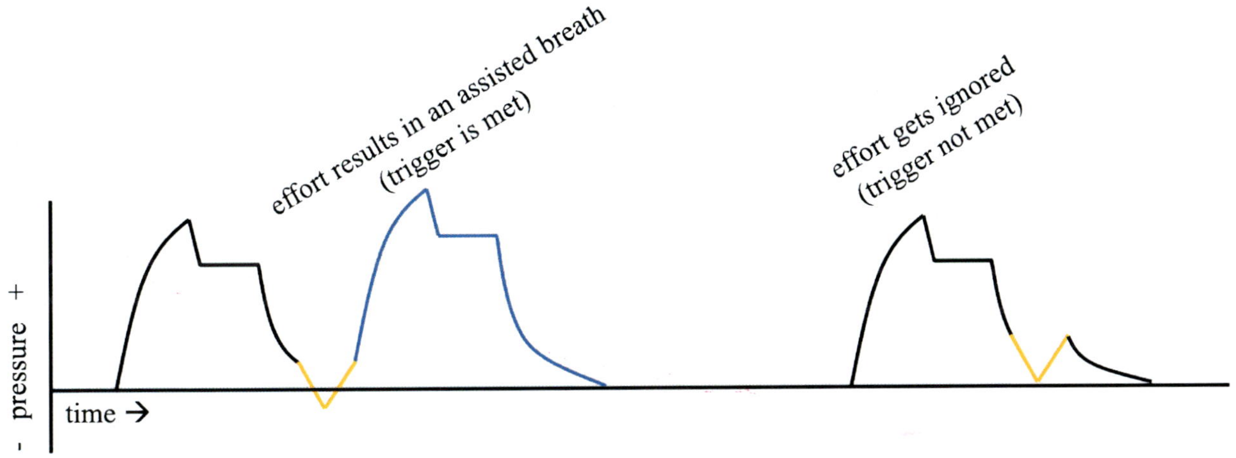

These yellow-effort situations do have the potential to cause harm, but they are less likely to result in breaths being delivered because of the ongoing breath that precedes them.[47] That harm comes from the increased pressure as a full breath is given before the prior one was completely done (left side, note the drift of maximum height on waveform). If the yellow effort doesn't result in a breath being delivered, this may cause some discomfort (right side, due to an expressed need that goes unaddressed), but that's probably OK. That said, a combination of green and yellow effort is just fine for our patients in assist control:

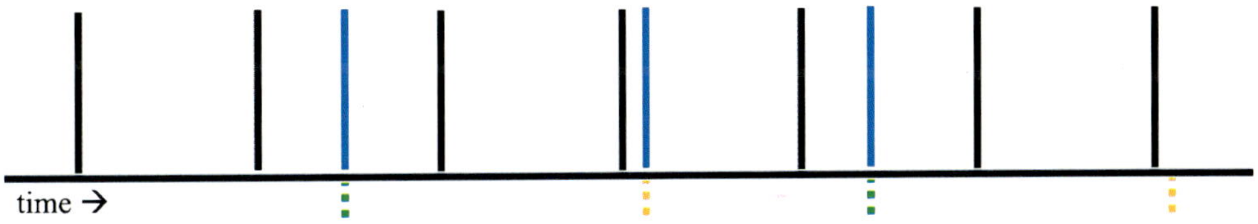

[47] Chatburn & friends, 2014 – There may also be a refractory period with some machines that prevents a subsequent trigger from occurring too soon after a breath has been given

AutoPEEP – intrinsic positive end-expiratory pressure; **OK** – alright

The issues with assist control begin when we get those red-effort situations in which a patient-triggered breath immediately precedes a time-triggered one:

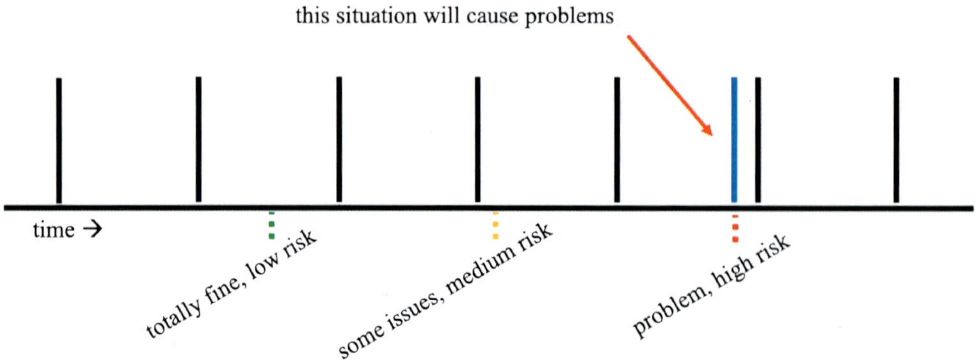

When this happens we get that same increase in pressure we just described (the drift of maximum height on the pressure waveform), but consistently and to a greater effect. As a waveform it would look like this:

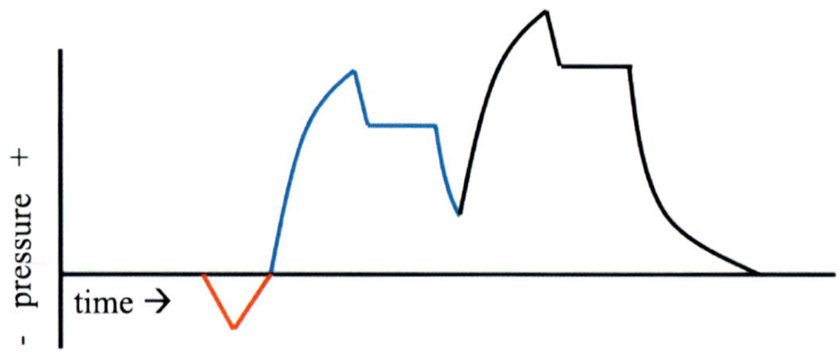

There is a complication known as **AutoPEEP**, or intrinsic positive end-expiratory pressure, in which this happens with some regularity resulting in sustained high pressures. AutoPEEP can also occur in assist control if we trigger a number of breaths in sequence. We'll revisit this idea again later, but here's how that might look (and we've left out colors and triggers for clarity):[48]

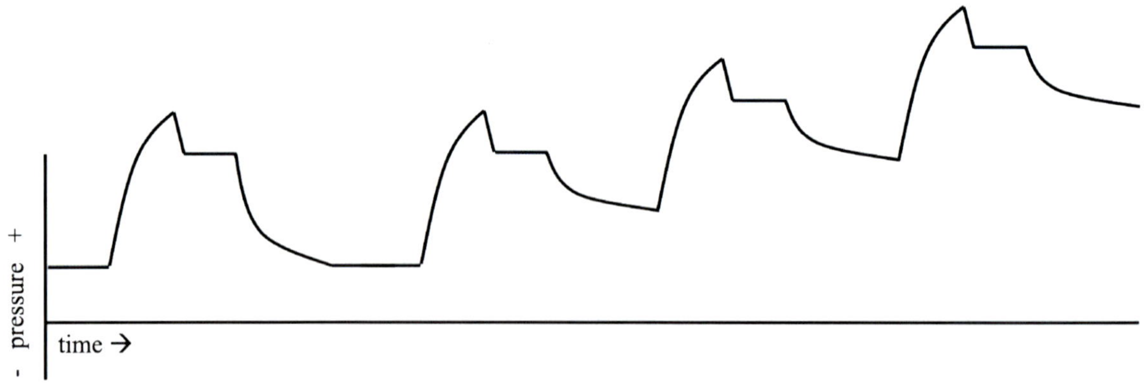

[48] In reality these stacked breaths will likely get cut short due to pressure limits we have set on the machine, but we'll explain that fully when we get to the section on **AutoPEEP**

PS – pressure support; **SIMV** – synchronized intermittent mandatory ventilation

So we've established that AutoPEEP can occur in assist control, but recognize that it doesn't always happen and that we can take proactive steps to make the mode safe for our patients. The primary benefit of assist control mode is that we can readily meet the patient's need for more volume using patient-triggered breaths. Another benefit is that it is predictable: patient effort that meets the trigger will get assisted to whatever parameter we have set into the machine. To say it another way, time-triggered and patient-triggered breaths will be the same. And then subjectively, assist control is easy to use. While this may not be the best reason to advocate its use in the field, it is simple to set up, easy to conceptualize, and when the primary complication of the mode does arise (AutoPEEP) there are specific actions we can take to fix it.[49]

To summarize, assist control delivers time-triggered breaths at a set rate and will supplement that with full breaths whenever a patient effort meets the trigger threshold. Upsides to this are that the increased needs of the patient are readily met, downsides are the risk for increased pressures and a move away from baseline (AutoPEEP, which we will get to later). As a general rule: anytime we have someone in assist control we need to be vigilant and monitor both airway pressures and AutoPEEP.

[49] And the specifics of how we both avoid and fix breath stacking will be discussed later, both in **AutoPEEP** and **Triggers**

AutoPEEP – intrinsic positive end-expiratory pressure; **OK** – alright

Synchronized Intermittent Mandatory Ventilation

Synchronized intermittent mandatory ventilation (SIMV) is an alternative mode of ventilation that seeks to mitigate the shortcomings of the more basic modes by using patient triggers, but has a mechanism built in that helps avoid the **AutoPEEP** complication of **Assist Control**. SIMV starts with the idea of mandatory breaths or a guaranteed number of time-triggered breaths to be given per minute. It then will support breaths taken in between these mandatory breaths. Furthermore, SIMV recognizes when patient effort is made in close proximity to a time-triggered, mandatory breath and assists that effort in a way similar to how breaths were assisted in assist control (i.e. a full breath is given). Now there are more differences between these various **Types of Breaths** and we'll get back to that eventually, but let's focus on the timing aspect of SIMV first. Going back to our original idea:

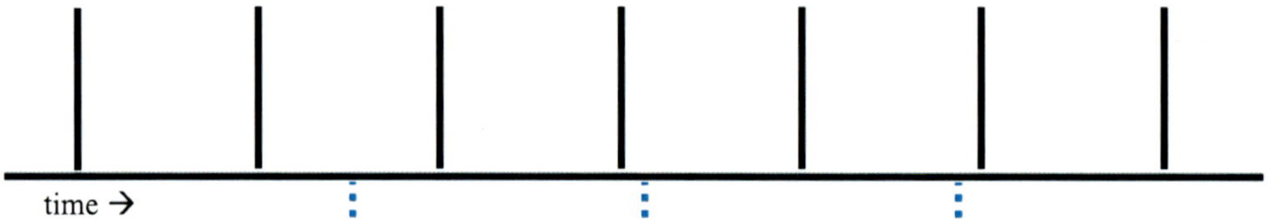

SIMV's method for determining how to handle the instances of patient effort is to break the timeline into two alternating categories: mandatory and spontaneous periods. If a patient trigger happens within a spontaneous period, it gets supported and that effort is facilitated by the machine in a manner that we will discuss soon;[50] if an effort occurs within a mandatory period it gets assisted, a full breath is delivered, and the breath that had been planned for that mandatory period gets skipped:[51]

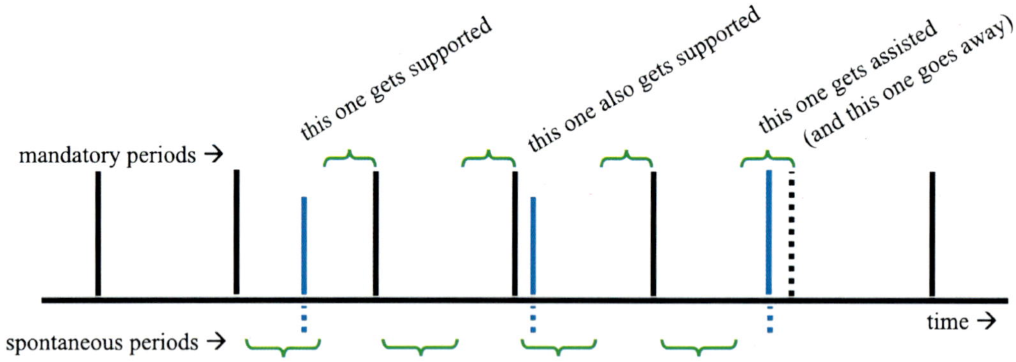

[50] Ollie, 2015 – This video explains the timing aspect of SIMV and how it was an improvement to intermittent mandatory ventilation (which we mentioned already in **Basic Modes of Ventilation** and will revisit again in just a moment)

[51] Wheeler & friends, 2008; Kumar, 2015 – The first explains this process of supporting a breath within the mandatory period as we've labeled it, the other is a brief overview that explains it using a different labeling system

PS – pressure support; **SIMV** – synchronized intermittent mandatory ventilation

To make sense of this graphic, we'll point out a few things. We are assuming that each instance of patient effort meets the trigger threshold to result in a breath. The difference in height of the blue lines is to distinguish supported breaths (smaller, left two) from assisted breaths (taller, right one). And that time-triggered breath at the far right gets omitted to avoid the AutoPEEP complication we saw in assist control.

As for the difference between supported breaths and assisted breaths: supported breaths only get a little bit of help from the machine and the assisted breaths are fully facilitated by the machine to a target amount of air, just as in assist control. Supported breaths are always supported via pressure, which helps the patient draw a breath a little bit easier; assisted breaths are carried out to meet specific goals by the machine based on settings we input and can be either volume-targeted or pressure-targeted (which we will expand on in the next section).[52] The practical difference is that pressure support breaths will give us a variable result that depends largely on the patient's contribution to that specific breath, while assisted breaths are more predictable.[53]

At the risk of getting ahead of ourselves, pressure support breaths are often expected to be less than or smaller than mandatory and assisted breaths (in terms of volume of air). While it may make sense to titrate pressure support up so that supported breaths match the other ones in this regard, it isn't quite as simple as increasing the pressure support value on the machine. That said, there is no reason that the volume of air in a pressure support breath should be less than the other ones, it's more an issue that it often just happens to turn out that way because of the details as to how these different **Types of Breaths** are brought into existence by the machine.[54]

And a few more things about SIMV mode: It originally came onto the scene as intermittent mandatory ventilation, which we already discussed. The "S" for synchronization was added when the mode was adapted to consider patient-triggers in close proximity to time-triggered breaths (i.e. breaths initiated by the patient within that mandatory period). The next improvement was pressure support to breaths triggered in the spontaneous period, so we sometimes see SIMV as we described it notated as SIMV + PS. To draw these all out: [55]

Intermittent Mandatory Ventilation

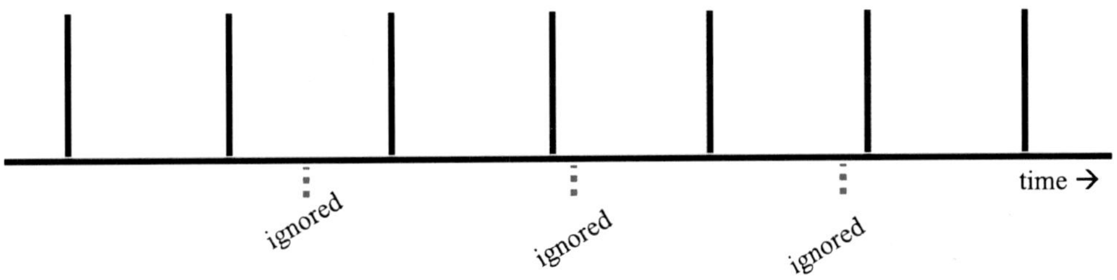

[52] Lodeserto, 2018 – This series provides an alternative explanation to this concept (i.e. how pressure support and pressure control breaths differ) and we will touch on it again in **Types of Breaths**

[53] Chatburn & friends, 2014 – And by convention both supported and assisted breaths could be labeled as assisted, it's just that pressure support breaths are a more specific type and we will discuss them that way just to remind readers about that difference

[54] Hess, 2005 – That said, the primary function of pressure support breaths is to relieve workload required by the patient and facilitate intrinsic respiratory effort, this is fundamentally different than a pressure control breath (discussed soon) in which we utilize pressure to deliver a breath regardless of patient effort; this article discusses how additional pressure support may not correlate as expected with an increase in **Tidal Volume** due to the way pressure support breaths are delivered

[55] Ghamloush & Hill, 2013 – We recognize that this confusion related to SIMV and its components is tough to follow, but navigate here for another explanation of how SIMV as we know it came to be

AutoPEEP – intrinsic positive end-expiratory pressure; **OK** – alright

SIMV (as it was known back in the day)

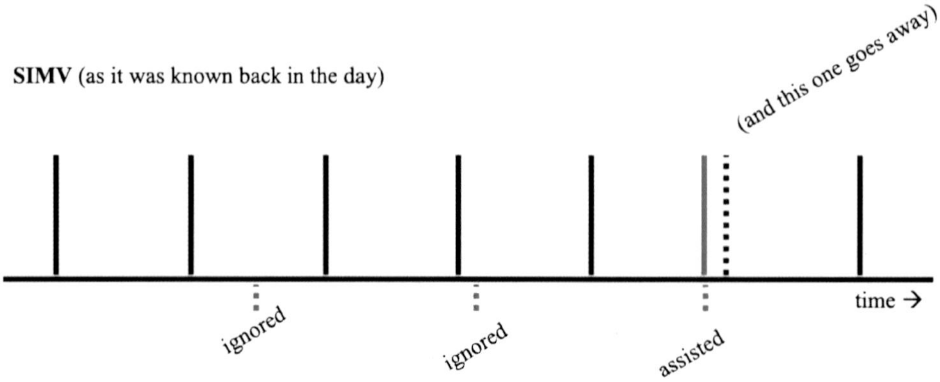

SIMV + PS (what we now refer to as SIMV)

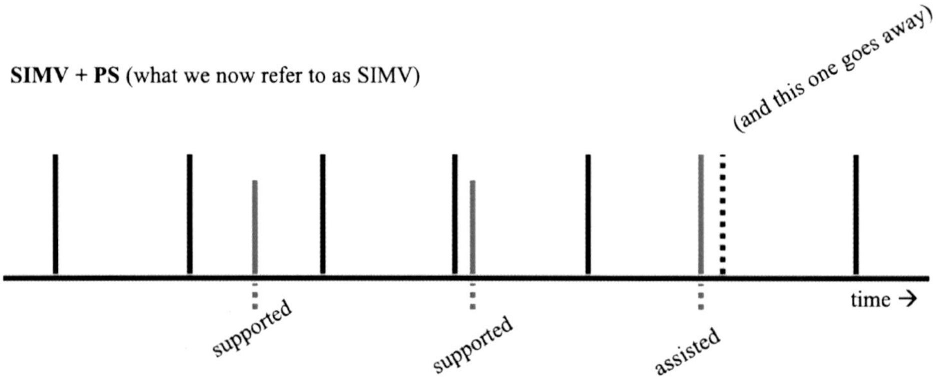

Another historical tidbit is that the mode was popularized as a method of weaning or getting someone transitioned from vent life to spontaneous breathing after an illness or intervention. The efficacy of SIMV for weaning has since been shown to be inferior to other methods. The result of all of this is that content on SIMV is often confounded by stuff that more accurately relates to intermittent mandatory ventilation or SIMV without pressure support and that draws conclusions from a concept (weaning) that doesn't much matter in the transport setting. Even though SIMV isn't used as often as it once was, it is important to understand that it does provide us with a valid alternative to assist control and both are legitimate choices in transport.

Now when we do put a patient on SIMV, there are some downsides to consider. First is that SIMV is less straightforward or intuitive than assist control. One component of this is that different breaths within the overall scheme may be delivered by different mechanisms and this can make it tough to manage settings when changes are warranted.[56] Another component is that supported breaths are harder to predict (in terms of volume), which may make it more difficult to meet a patient's need for more air. It can also be tough for us to align machine effort with patient effort (i.e. SIMV is more prone to asynchrony).[57] And last thing, which may or may not be a valid reason in and of itself, SIMV is less common than assist control mode. This means that exposure to and experience with the mode is likely less and also that patient handoffs may not be as fluid as they would be if the patient were in assist control.

---

[56] We will talk further about these **Types of Breaths** in a later section, but this particular source of confusion is when we have someone in SIMV and **Volume Control**; in these cases some breaths are given by volume and others are given by pressure
[57] We will discuss this idea of ventilator synchrony in **Comfort**

PS – pressure support; SIMV – synchronized intermittent mandatory ventilation

To summarize, SIMV is a mode that both supports patient effort to breathe via pressure support breaths and avoids breath stacking by not delivering breaths in close proximity to others. This avoids the problem of AutoPEEP that we discussed in regard to assist control. On the other hand, SIMV has been associated with ventilator asynchrony and can be harder to both conceptualize and monitor than assist control ventilation (due to the different types of breaths involved). All that said, SIMV is an appropriate mode to use in transport and provides clinicians with an alternative to assist control.

And Beyond…

Now that we know about both assist control and SIMV modes, the decision becomes which mode to use for a given patient. While many folks have their preference and we could argue one over the other all day long until we are both blue in the face, the bottom line is that either mode could work for just about any patient type. Here's the general strategy we'll recommend (and we will revisit this idea at the very end when we talk about building out a guideline and putting it all together): if we have a patient already on the vent and all is well, just stick with whichever mode they are working with; if we are starting from scratch or reworking the settings altogether, try what our machine defaults to and then change modes if we need to down the line. That's about as simple as we can make it. All that said, there are cases in which one mode may be preferred over another and we will talk about those as they come up.

cmH_2O – centimeters of water; **ml** – milliliter; **OK** – alright; **PRVC** – pressure-regulated volume control

Control of Ventilation

The next decision is to choose whether we want to control volume or pressure. If we choose to control volume, airway pressure will function as the dependent variable (i.e. we won't be able to directly control it); if we choose to control pressure, volume will function as the dependent variable. There is no right or wrong answer to this dilemma, but the general trend is that we use volume control in most cases and pressure control with pediatrics or when we are especially concerned about airway pressures.[58] Not saying this is the best decision, just saying that's how it's been done.

The reason for this is twofold. First (and arguably most relevant), the machines tend to default to volume control unless we do something to intentionally get out of it. Second, volume control is a bit easier for some folks to wrap their heads around. It's a little more intuitive to think about set volumes and resultant pressures than it is the other way. But as we said above, there is no right or wrong; we can just as effectively and safely ventilate a baby in volume control as we can an adult in pressure control (even though this is contrary to what we normally do), as long as we know the underlaying concepts and keep an eye on all the important things along the way!

[58] Kneyber & friends, 2017 – Note that even the people who make the rules on pediatric ventilation don't endorse one method of control over another…

cmH_2O – centimeters of water; **ml** – milliliter; **OK** – alright; **PRVC** – pressure-regulated volume control

Volume Control

In volume control ventilation we choose how much volume we want to push down the circuit with each breath delivered.[59] This tidal volume that we put in goes to the lungs, does its thing at the alveolar level, and then gets exhaled out of the circuit. When we say tidal volume we are referring to the air going into the system from the machine; those other two concepts (alveolar tidal volume and exhaled tidal volume) vary from that value due to a number of different factors. Let's see how this looks in a graphic and then we'll hash out the details:

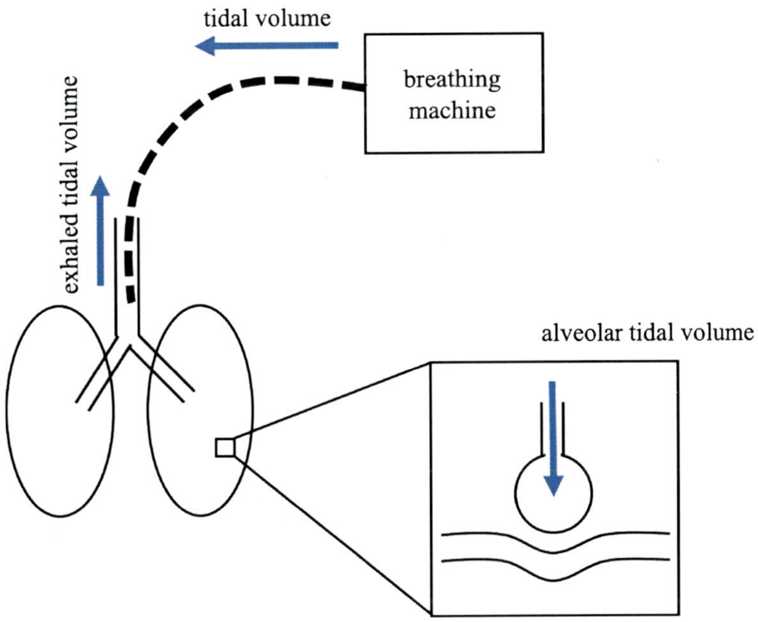

[59] To say it another way, in volume control we control **Tidal Volume** directly – a concept we mention here and then discuss again in much more detail in the near future

cmH_2O – centimeters of water; **ml** – milliliter; **OK** – alright; **PRVC** – pressure-regulated volume control

Exhaled tidal volume is generally about the same as tidal volume, but after some air is lost to the vent circuit and/ or to the tissues in the respiratory system. This results in the potential to overestimate volume delivered, which becomes particularly important with smaller volumes of air (i.e. pediatrics).[60] And alveolar tidal volume is exhaled tidal volume minus anatomic dead space. Recognizing the fact that not all of that alveolar tidal volume will always participate in gas exchange due to the idea of alveolar dead space, the volume of air that makes it to the alveoli is about two-thirds of what we push into the system.[61] Here's how it all looks:

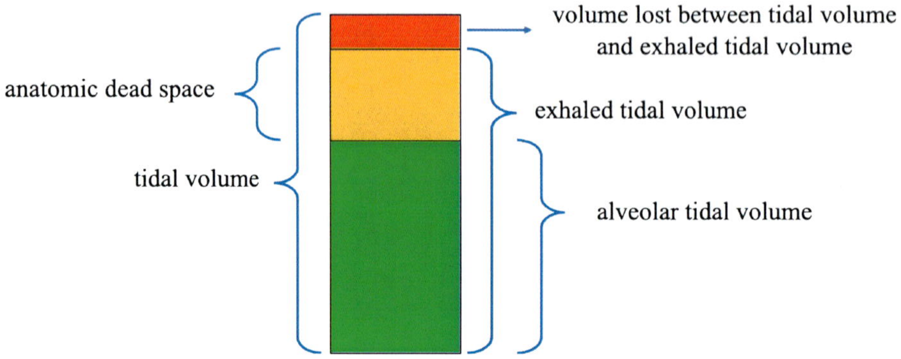

While alveolar tidal volume seems a few steps removed from the tidal volume we set on the machine, volume control ventilation allows us to control alveolar tidal volume as directly as possible. The result of that, however, is an increase in pressure that is dependent on the amount of air we set and how that air moves through the respiratory system. For now we will defer a discussion of how we describe this air movement (i.e. its speed or flow), just know that pushing a preset volume in means that pressure changes happen as a result of that air movement and that certain pressure changes (i.e. too much air too fast) can cause damage to the alveoli.[62] While the alveoli do expand with added volume, at a certain point we can overinflate them. This results in what we call barotrauma and we for sure want to avoid that.

[60] We talked about this overestimation of air delivered already in **Dead Space** and will address it again in the **Appendix**

[61] Yartsev, 2019 – This idea that alveolar tidal volume is about two-thirds of delivered tidal volume gets a bit more complicated, but we'll get back to it in **Ventilation**; for now take a look at the linked webpage for more on the idea

[62] Flowers & friends, 2019 – As another example of Gas Laws in action, this process is partly described by Boyle's Law (pressure change as a result of volume increase)

cmH₂O – centimeters of water; **ml** – milliliter; **OK** – alright; **PRVC** – pressure-regulated volume control

We will get more into all of these concepts later, but a high pressure in volume control can be due to alveoli inflated beyond their capacity, some restriction to the expansion of the chest wall, or decreased air movement through the airways:

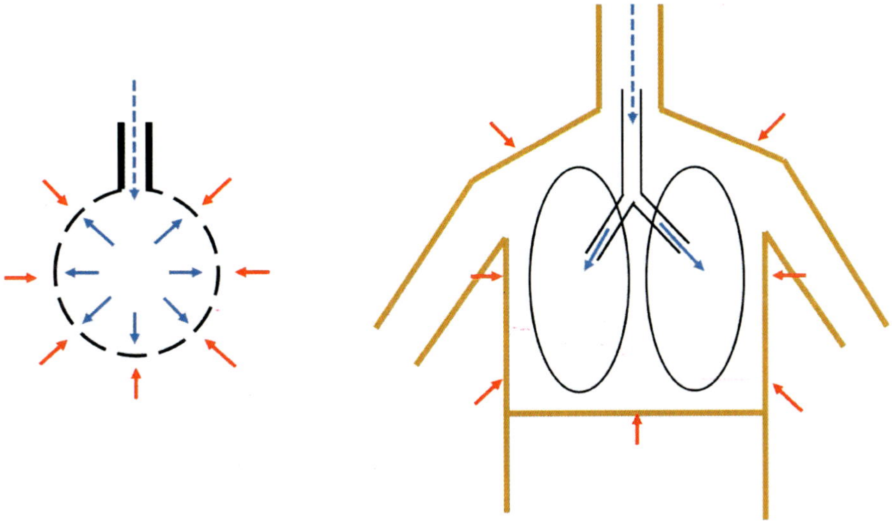

The risk we face in volume control ventilation is that we can injure the alveoli or cause barotrauma when they are overinflated, as shown above on the left. To say this another way: there are three distinct reasons why we may see high pressures and one of those three, overdistended alveoli, is our area of concern in this discussion. We avoid this by monitoring airway pressures and adjusting the volume input to avoid causing damage.[63] We will get to the specifics as to how we do that eventually, for now it's OK to leave it as so: in volume control ventilation we control the amount of air going into the circuit at the expense of control over resultant pressures. That said, we always need to monitor airway pressures during volume control ventilation in order to avoid causing damage to the alveoli. In addition, volume control lends itself to an overestimation of alveolar tidal volume if we forget to factor in dead space.

[63] While there are other parameters that we can adjust to avoid higher pressures (which we will get to later), it helps to simplify things this way: more volume = more pressure

cmH_2O – centimeters of water; **ml** – milliliter; **OK** – alright; **PRVC** – pressure-regulated volume control

Pressure Control

In the other corner of the arena we have pressure control ventilation.[64] In this system, a breath happens as so: we have a dialed-in pressure, the machine spins up to maintain that pressure, the air all the way from machine to alveoli equalize to this pressure for an amount of time, then the breath cycles off and we go back to baseline. Because our input here is pressure, volume becomes our dependent variable (exhaled tidal volume, to be exact and as we noted before).[65] Let's draw it out and see if we can make it a little clearer:

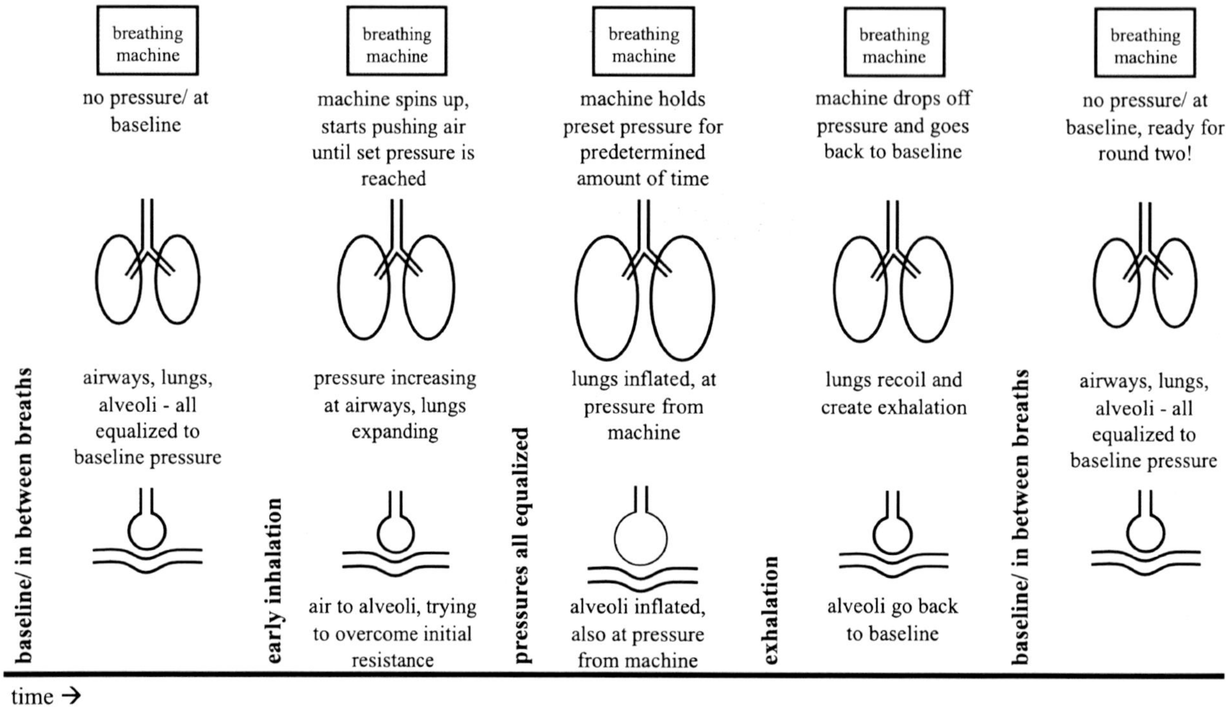

In the fourth column, we see that recoil of the lungs (a passive exhalation) occurs when the pressure that had been keeping those lungs inflated drops off. This volume of air that gets pushed out of the circuit as the lungs fall back to baseline is our exhaled tidal volume. We then have to actively observe to make sure this volume meets the goal we have in mind for what volume this patient ought to be getting with each breath delivered. If this exhaled tidal volume is not what we want it to be, then we adjust the pressure in the system to get closer to our goal: more pressure means more volume, less pressure means less volume.

---

[64] Meeks, 2018; Yartsev, 2019 – And we phrased it this way because there is much debate out there in vent world as to which strategy (volume or pressure) is superior; see referenced podcast and article for more information

[65] And if a machine is capable of pressure control ventilation it will surely have a mechanism for measuring exhaled tidal volume; in the previous section we noted that some machines don't give us this value, but those machines tend to do volume control ventilation only

cmH_2O – centimeters of water; **ml** – milliliter; **OK** – alright; **PRVC** – pressure-regulated volume control

One thing worth pointing out here is that in pressure control ventilation we don't have to bother with considering that flexibility or stretch that we discussed when we talked about dead space (i.e. the compliance of the vent circuit), as the only way we have to measure volume is via exhaled tidal volume or what the patient breathes out (which is downstream of all that flexing). We do still need to consider anatomic and alveolar dead space, just as we did with volume control, but the stretch factor we introduce in our circuit is eliminated. This is a big advantage of pressure control ventilation with small patients: forgetting to factor in 10ml (arbitrary number) in an adult is no big deal, forgetting to do so for a baby with small tidal volumes is huge.[66]

Another benefit of pressure control is that we avoid the risk of over-inflation or high pressures at the alveolar level. The highest pressure those alveoli will see is whatever value we program into the machine.[67] As long as we follow some basic guidelines as to what a safe pressure is, there's not much risk of harm or barotrauma. The downside is that we don't have as good of control (compared to volume control) over the amount or volume of air that we are putting into the system; instead we have to continually monitor exhaled tidal volumes and adjust to our goals.[68]

To summarize: in pressure control ventilation we control the pressure put into the system at the expense of control over resultant volumes. That said, we always need to monitor those volumes when we have a patient in pressure control in order to avoid hyper- or hypoventilation. In addition, pressure control ventilation makes it a little more difficult to manage ventilation (as opposed to oxygenation – again, concepts we will get to later on), due to the breath to breath variability in volumes.[69] The big advantage of pressure control is that we avoid the high pressures that can result from volume control.[70]

[66] We will address the idea of how volume control can lead to an overestimation of actual volume delivered (and how pressure control can mitigate that) in the **Appendix**

[67] While it is generally true that the value dialed in for pressure control is the highest pressure the system will see as a breath is delivered, there are some exceptions that we'll chat about in **Airway Pressures in Pressure Control?**

[68] Ashworth & friends, 2018 – Refer to this article for a much more detailed discussion of how we can work towards our ventilation goals in pressure control ventilation

[69] And to skip ahead and look at these sections, link to them here: **Ventilation** and **Oxygenation**

[70] There are more advantages to pressure control ventilation (such as how pressure control breaths differ from volume control ones in regard to flow waveforms), but we'll get to that stuff later on in **Types of Breaths**

cmH_2O – centimeters of water; **ml** – milliliter; **OK** – alright; **PRVC** – pressure-regulated volume control

Pressure-Regulated Volume Control

Pressure-regulated volume control (PRVC) is one attempt to get at the best of both worlds when it comes to this volume versus pressure conundrum. In this type of ventilation we dial in a goal for tidal volume and put an upper limit on pressure, then the machine tries to give breaths to the goal volume using the lowest possible pressure and without exceeding the limit we have set.[71] The machine makes adjustments to how it delivers each breath by looking at previous breaths and adjusting delivery to add or take away volume working towards the preset tidal volume goal. In the event that it can't reach the goal volume without exceeding the upper pressure limit, volume is sacrificed – think of the pressure regulated part as a hard stop.

Let's visualize this over a few breaths to see what it would look like:

goal tidal volume: 400ml
pressure cap: $30cmH_2O$

breath one	**breath two**	**breath three**	**breath four**	**breath five**	**breath six**
initial breath	more pressure	a little less pressure	same pressure	a little more pressure	same pressure
$25cmH_2O$	$30cmH_2O$	$28cmH_2O$	$28cmH_2O$	$29cmH_2O$	$29cmH_2O$
300ml	450ml	400ml	375ml	400ml	400ml

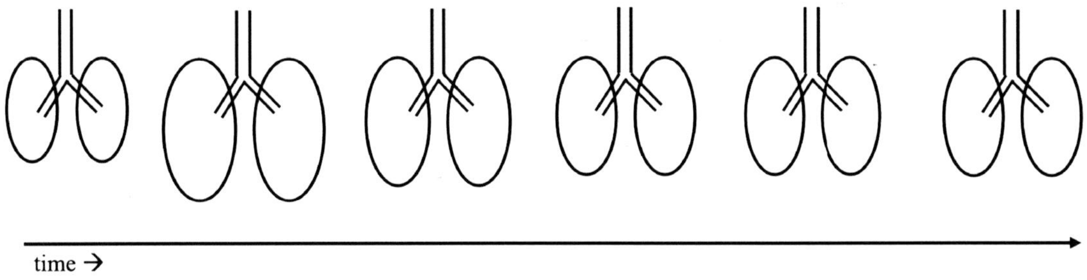

We can also think of this in an algorithmic fashion where the machine decides where each breath ends up in relation to our goal and then adjusts the subsequent breath in a cyclical manner:

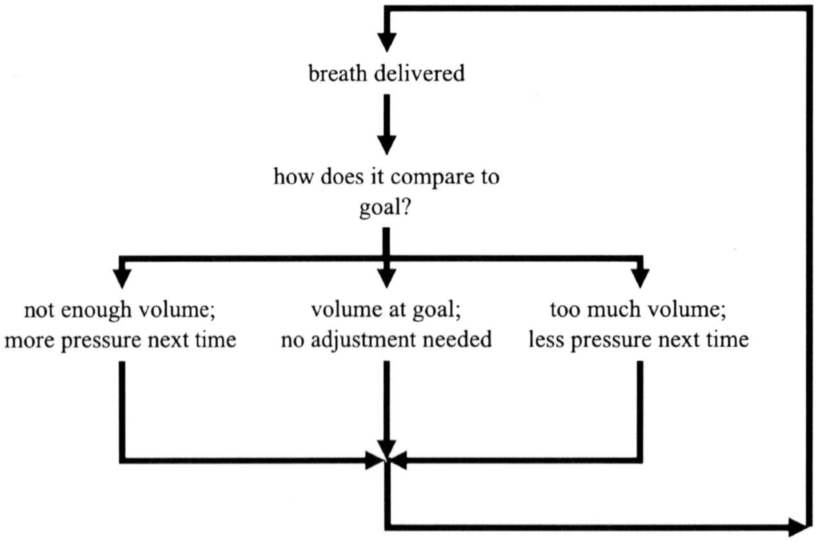

[71] In the first graphic on this page and moving forward we call this pressure limit in a PRVC breath the pressure cap for lack of a better term, but we will discuss it more in just a moment

cmH_2O – centimeters of water; **ml** – milliliter; **OK** – alright; **PRVC** – pressure-regulated volume control

This mechanism of decision making one breath at a time doesn't quite describe the process accurately, but it gives the right idea. In reality, the machine looks back at the last few breaths and builds a small data set from which it decides how to deliver the next breath. So the system is more refined than our crude representation.

To flush out a few more details on this PRVC concept, let's look at another example of a few consecutive breaths. In this example, breaths fall under goal (in terms of volume). The result of this would be a drop in minute volume or air moved per unit time.[72] It's important to keep this in mind with PRVC, as we can inadvertently lose some minute volume in an effort to avoid high pressures:

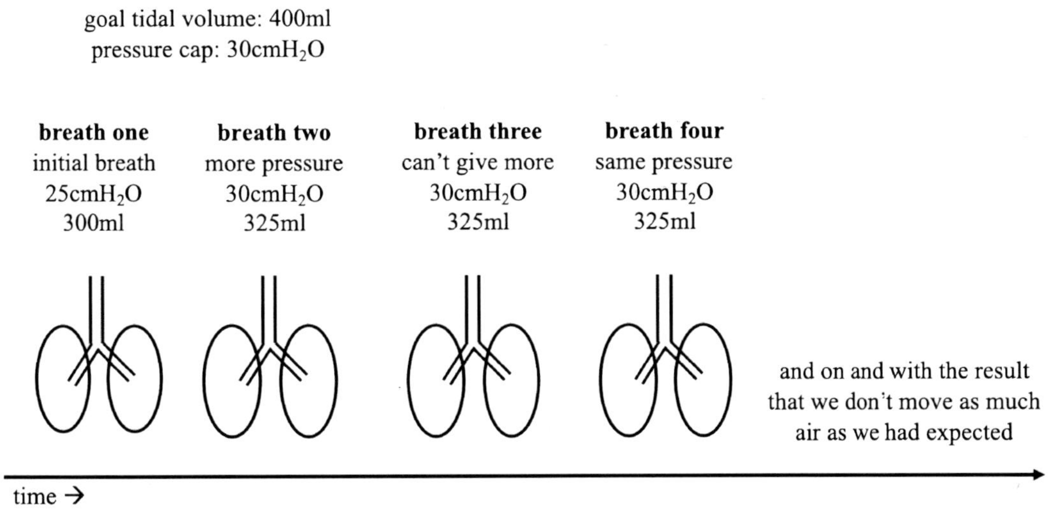

A few more things about PRVC: pressure cap is a make-believe term and the machine most often uses $5cmH_20$ less than the set high-pressure limit for this value.[73] There are also restrictions on how much variation occurs from one breath to the next. To say it another way, the machine won't make drastic changes in response to one or two funky breaths. Another thing: the machine has a system to get this whole process started by giving test breaths via different methods when it first gets set up.[74] Along that same idea, the machine doesn't know how much air (i.e. **Tidal Volume**) it gives with each breath until after the fact when it sees the exhaled tidal volume, that's why it can overshoot the goal. Last thing: PRVC is good when we are worried about barotrauma or giving too much pressure, but it is important to make sure we keep an eye on volumes delivered and compare it to our calculated goal.

---

[72] This concept of **Minute Volume** is discussed in much more detail in just a few sections

[73] And limits are discussed later when we get to **Alarms**

[74] Maher, 2019 – Short video that describes this idea of test breaths and gives a brief overview of PRVC (and it is just one video is a large series, so take a look at the rest of his content for more)

cmH_2O – centimeters of water; **FiO_2** – fraction of inspired oxygen; **IBW** – ideal body weight; **I:E** – inspiratory to expiratory; **I-time** – inspiratory time; **kg** – kilogram; **LPM** – liters per minute; **min** – minute; **ml** – milliliter; **mmHg** – millimeters of mercury

Vent Parameters, Round One

The next step on our journey is to explain the ins and outs of some of the terms we use to describe different aspects of ventilation. Some of these have been mentioned already (and a few discussed in detail), but most of the complete explanations have been left out up until this point in an effort to better organize thoughts in a linear, stepwise fashion. If it helps to go back to previous sections after this discussion, go for it. Also, keep in mind that this is not an exhaustive list of all the terms, these are just the basics and more will come later.

Tidal Volume

Tidal volume is the amount of air moved in a given breath. As previously discussed, it helps to break this concept up into two distinct terms: tidal volume and exhaled tidal volume.[75] Tidal volume, in this way of thinking, would be the volume of air we put into the system, while exhaled tidal volume would be the volume of air that comes out of the system. Tidal volume may be notated as TV or Vt; exhaled tidal volume is notated as Vte.

Tidal volume varies with the size of the patient and the normal range is 6-8ml/kg of **Ideal Body Weight**. Recall the discussion we already had about IBW and the idea that lung size is best correlated to height. Also recognize that 6-8ml/kg IBW is just a framework from which we start when determining our initial settings and that tidal volume can range from 4-12ml/kg IBW, depending on the specific situation that we are up against.[76] We will talk further on that when we get into ventilator strategies.

And just to recap what we already discussed, add in some values, and then demonstrate it again in a slightly different way:

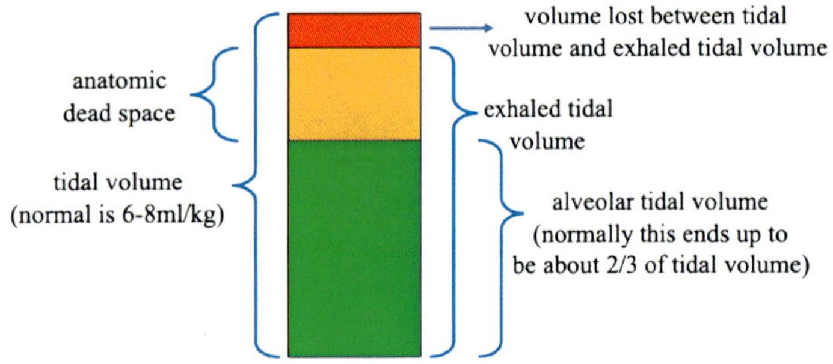

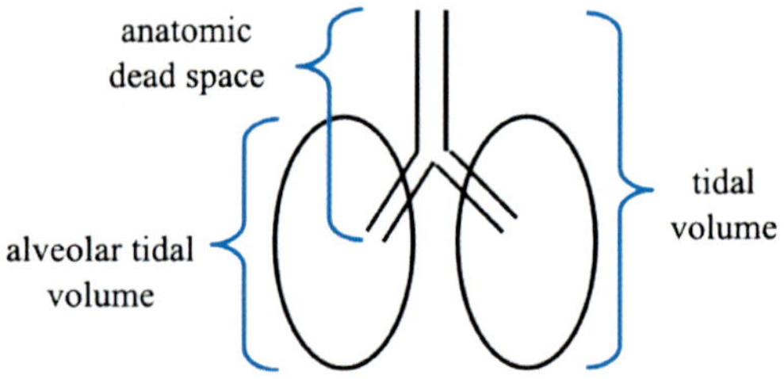

[75] Tidal volume and exhaled tidal volume were first discussed back in **Volume Control**

[76] Davies & friends, 2016 – These guys offer a much more in-depth discussion about this idea of having a preset tidal volume goal for all patient populations and why we should or shouldn't deviate from that framework in our vent management

MV – minute volume; **OK** – alright; **PALS** – pediatric advanced life support; **PEEP** – positive end-expiratory pressure; **PSI** – pounds per square inch; **RR** – respiratory rate; **s** – second; **TV** – tidal volume

One more thing to mention here. We have a quantity of air in that last graphic labeled "volume lost between tidal volume and exhaled tidal volume" and this is generally an OK assumption to make (as we discussed before in **Volume Control**), but it isn't always the case because exhaled tidal volume can sometimes exceed tidal volume for various reasons. For example, there may be some breath to breath variation with the spontaneously breathing patient or (s)he may forcibly exhale after a breath is given. There is also the idea that cold air from the supply or machine end of the system will warm and expand as it enters the airways and lungs.[77] These are just a few examples, we just wanted to point out that exhaled tidal volume doesn't always have to be less that tidal volume and that reasons for this vary widely.

[77] Flowers & friends, 2019 – This idea of cold air expanding with an increase in temperature would be an example of Charles' Law

cmH$_2$O – centimeters of water; **FiO$_2$** – fraction of inspired oxygen; **IBW** – ideal body weight; **I:E** – inspiratory to expiratory; **I-time** – inspiratory time; **kg** – kilogram; **LPM** – liters per minute; **min** – minute; **ml** – milliliter; **mmHg** – millimeters of mercury

Respiratory Rate

Respiratory rate (RR) describes how many breaths are delivered and/ or taken in one minute. While rate is often considered the value we put into the machine and frequency (f) is the total number of breaths per minute after patient-triggered breaths are considered, we will use respiratory rate, or simply rate, to describe this concept as a whole moving forward. With that said, know that if we want to decrease rate and the patient is triggering breaths spontaneously, decreasing rate on the vent won't have the intended effect. No need to dwell on that idea now, we'll come back to it later on.[78]

Normal parameters vary by age, but the typical adult rate is 12-20 and pediatric rates are as outlined on our Broselow Tape[79] or by this chart from the PALS Manual:[80]

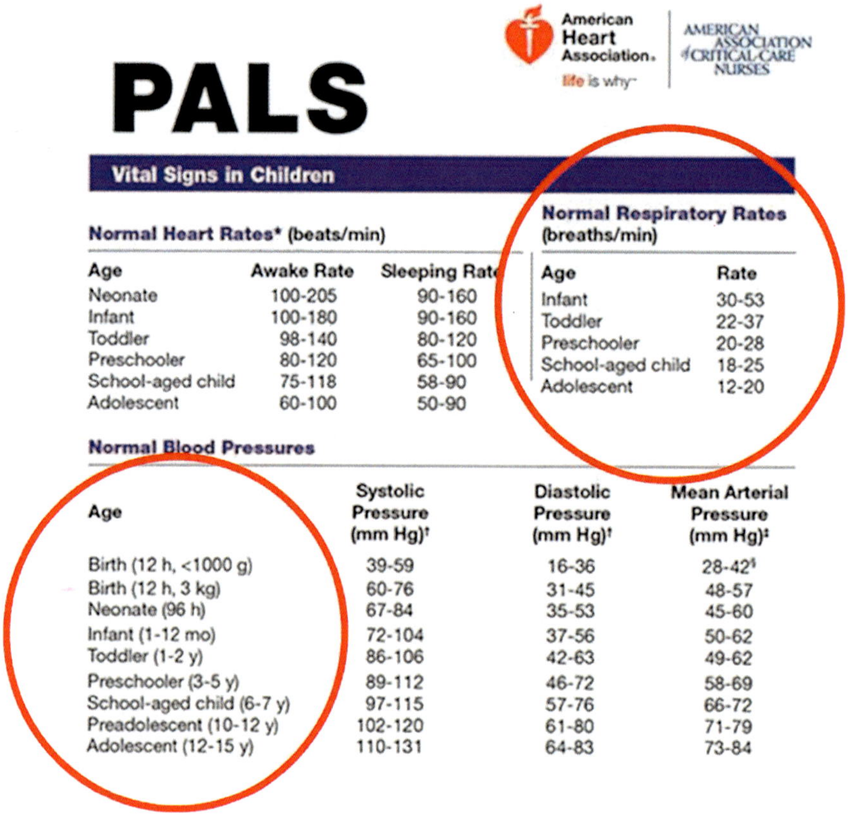
American Heart Association. life is why
AMERICAN ASSOCIATION of CRITICAL-CARE NURSES

PALS

Vital Signs in Children

Normal Heart Rates* (beats/min)

Age	Awake Rate	Sleeping Rate
Neonate	100-205	90-160
Infant	100-180	90-160
Toddler	98-140	80-120
Preschooler	80-120	65-100
School-aged child	75-118	58-90
Adolescent	60-100	50-90

Normal Respiratory Rates (breaths/min)

Age	Rate
Infant	30-53
Toddler	22-37
Preschooler	20-28
School-aged child	18-25
Adolescent	12-20

Normal Blood Pressures

Age	Systolic Pressure (mm Hg)†	Diastolic Pressure (mm Hg)†	Mean Arterial Pressure (mm Hg)‡
Birth (12 h, <1000 g)	39-59	16-36	28-42§
Birth (12 h, 3 kg)	60-76	31-45	48-57
Neonate (96 h)	67-84	35-53	45-60
Infant (1-12 mo)	72-104	37-56	50-62
Toddler (1-2 y)	86-106	42-63	49-62
Preschooler (3-5 y)	89-112	46-72	58-69
School-aged child (6-7 y)	97-115	57-76	66-72
Preadolescent (10-12 y)	102-120	61-80	71-79
Adolescent (12-15 y)	110-131	64-83	73-84

---

[78] This concept of an observed respiratory rate being greater than a set rate and what we can do about it is discussed in **Overbreathing**
[79] Kindig & friends, 2019 – This article gives a good overview of all the features newer Broselow Tapes have to offer, to include initial vent settings that roughly approximate the ones we discuss in this section
[80] American Heart Association, 2016 (image) - As a quick disclaimer: these normal respiratory rates as outlined in PALS are not intended to be used for determining vent settings, rather they are outlined as such to identify normal and abnormal findings in an assessment; with that said, most transport clinicians are familiar with this reference and have ready access to it, so it makes sense to build our concept of vent management from a known source rather than introduce new values and numbers with which we may not be familiar

MV – minute volume; **OK** – alright; **PALS** – pediatric advanced life support; **PEEP** – positive end-expiratory pressure; **PSI** – pounds per square inch; **RR** – respiratory rate; **s** – second; **TV** – tidal volume

For the detail-oriented people out there, there are some data points missing from this PALS chart. One strategy would be to guess based on available data (i.e. no listed rate for a 9-year-old, but we could assume a value that falls in between the school-aged child range and that for adolescents). Another option is to use this chart we've put together based on the existing data in the PALS chart:[81]

age description	**age (years)**	**rate**
infant	.083 (1 month) – 1	30 – 53
toddler	1 – 2	22 – 37
preschooler	3 – 5	22 – 28
school-aged child	6 – 7	18 – 25
big kid	8 – 9	17 – 25
preadolescent	10 – 12	14 – 23
adolescent	12 – 15	12 – 20
adult	16 and up	12 – 20

Last thing: there are times that we set rate above or below what might be considered normal for the patient's age, but we'll get to those specifics when we discuss vent strategies for different situations later on.

[81] See **Appendix** for a discussion of how this chart to outline normal respiratory rate values by age was created

cmH₂O – centimeters of water; **FiO₂** – fraction of inspired oxygen; **IBW** – ideal body weight; **I:E** – inspiratory to expiratory; **I-time** – inspiratory time; **kg** – kilogram; **LPM** – liters per minute; **min** – minute; **ml** – milliliter; **mmHg** – millimeters of mercury

Minute Volume

Minute volume (MV), also known as minute ventilation (VE), is the amount of air moved in one full minute. It is the product of **Tidal Volume** and **Respiratory Rate**:

$$MV = RR \times TV$$

Minute volume is the primary mechanism by which we control **Ventilation**. We will discuss soon how to manipulate both tidal volume and rate to address ventilation in just a bit, so don't worry about that for the moment. A normal minute volume for the adult patient is often cited at 4 – 8 liters per minute (LPM), but we prefer to use a weight-based calculation so that it applies to all patient sizes:[82]

$$MV \approx 100ml/kg\ IBW/min$$

We've chosen to represent that minute volume is roughly (≈) 100ml/kg IBW/min because that goal is less of a hard-set requirement than a guideline by which we initiate ventilation in most cases. For the majority of patients this calculated value will be adequate, but there are times in which we ought to aim above or below for various reasons. For example, with both pediatric patients and those with **Acidosis**, we will aim higher than that; with others we may tolerate a minute volume below that value by way of a concept known as permissive hypercapnia.[83] We will eventually get into the details on how we go about making that decision for different patient types, but for now we'll leave it at that.

There can be different types of minute volume, just as there were with tidal volume. Minute volume or minute ventilation typically describes what we dial into the machine, then we tag exhaled on to either term (abbreviated MVe) to describe feedback the machine gives us about what the patient breathes out. Lastly there is alveolar minute ventilation (VA) which takes out anatomic dead space from the equation. While alveolar minute volume (another way of describing minute ventilation) is an important concept to consider, we base initial goals and calculations on minute volume or exhaled minute volume and not on alveolar ventilation.[84]

[82] Weingart, 2010; Yartsev, 2019 – These guys cite a goal minute volume for the intubated patient as 120ml/kg/min and 70-110ml/kg/min, respectively; we've opted to go with 100ml/kg/min as a starting point due to ease of calculations and simplicity
[83] Pruitt, 2007 – We cite this again later when we discuss both the **Obstruction** and **Lung Injury** strategies, but it outlines the idea of this permissive hypercapnia approach to certain patient populations
[84] We do, however, make subsequent changes to address ventilation with these alveolar volumes in mind and we will get to that in **Ventilation**

MV – minute volume; **OK** – alright; **PALS** – pediatric advanced life support; **PEEP** – positive end-expiratory pressure; **PSI** – pounds per square inch; **RR** – respiratory rate; **s** – second; **TV** – tidal volume

Fraction of Inspired Oxygen

Fraction of inspired oxygen (FiO_2) describes the amount of oxygen in the mix of gasses that we push into the patient's vent circuit when we give a breath. 100% oxygen would be an FiO_2 of 1.0; 21% oxygen or ambient air would be an FiO_2 of 0.21. Adjusting FiO_2 is often the easiest way we can address an **Oxygenation** issue, but we'll discuss fixing things in just a little while. FiO_2 is typically a parameter we dial in directly to the machine, but it can also be calculated based on how much oxygen we put into the machine and how much total air the machine puts out:[85]

$$FiO_2 = \text{total amount of oxygen} \div \text{total amount of air}$$

and then we can use the concept of flow to quantify these values in this equation:[86]

assume 10LPM of oxygen going in
and 60LPM of total flow

$$FiO_2 = [(10LPM \times 100\%) + (50LPM \times 21\%)] \div 60LPM$$
$$FiO_2 = 34\% \text{ or } 0.34$$

Now there is never really a need to do this sort of calculation, as the machine will allow us to bypass the math and directly provide a chosen FiO_2 as long as our oxygen source is adequate (such as one of those 50PSI adapters like we see on the wall of the ambulance or hospital). And if we do bypass that mechanism by using a low-flow oxygen source (i.e. normal oxygen tubing), each manufacturer has different recommendations as to how we should estimate an FiO_2 based on the settings we have dialed in and the flow of oxygen into the system.

[85] Reading, 2016 – For more detail on this type of calculation to determine an FiO_2 algebraically, take a look at this article

[86] And we won't talk about flow in depth until **Types of Breaths**

Positive End-Expiratory Pressure

Positive end-expiratory pressure (PEEP) describes the positive pressure that remains in the alveoli at the end of expiration. And let's recognize that we basically explained a term using the words it's made up of, so we'll try it another way via a few steps. During mechanical ventilation we push air into the alveoli on inspiration, then that air moves out of the alveoli on expiration. We tend to conceptualize this as a net-zero movement of air where the alveoli go from deflated to inflated and then back to deflated, as so:

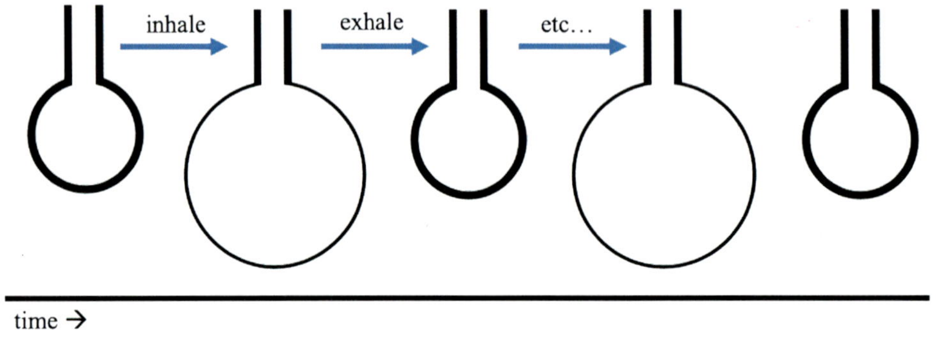

The truth is that we can put pressure into the alveoli and then maintain it throughout exhalation (in the form of PEEP). So rather than the alveolar air sac deflating all the way back to its original size, it deflates only part way:

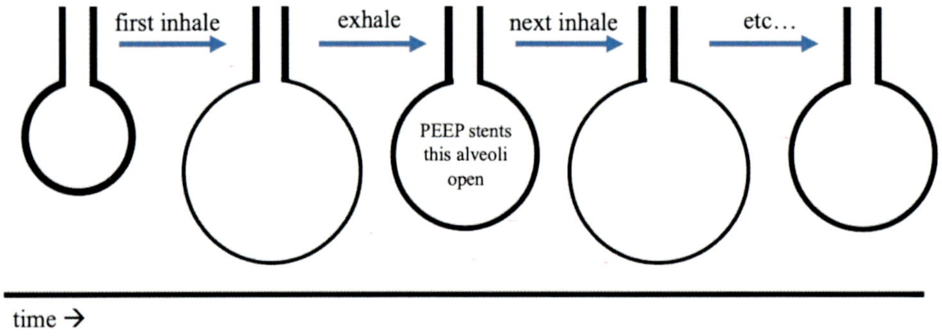

MV – minute volume; **OK** – alright; **PALS** – pediatric advanced life support; **PEEP** – positive end-expiratory pressure; **PSI** – pounds per square inch; **RR** – respiratory rate; **s** – second; **TV** – tidal volume

Recall from our previous discussion of **Alveolar Surface Area** that the more inflated the alveoli are, the more they can participate in gas exchange. This is due to both more surface area and a thinner membrane across which gasses must diffuse.[87] Next, add to that the idea that blood flow though the pulmonary capillary bed is continuous, it doesn't stop when inhalation stops. This means that pulmonary respiration or gas exchange across the alveolar membrane occurs throughout the respiratory cycle, both on inhale and exhale. PEEP helps facilitate this gas process on the exhalation side and then makes it easier to further maximize the effect during inhalation (i.e. a better starting point from which inhalation begins).

Another idea particularly relevant to this discussion of PEEP is that the stenting or opening-up of alveoli doesn't always happen in one breath as it's been depicted in the above drawing. Sometimes it takes time to get from that left-most, deflated stage to a recruited or opened-up stage. Part of the reason for that is that there is fluid around the surface of the alveoli that resists expansion. Think of it as molecules on the alveolar surface that are holding hands with one another; as we increase the size of the alveoli, we increase the distance between those hand-holders and make expansion easier:

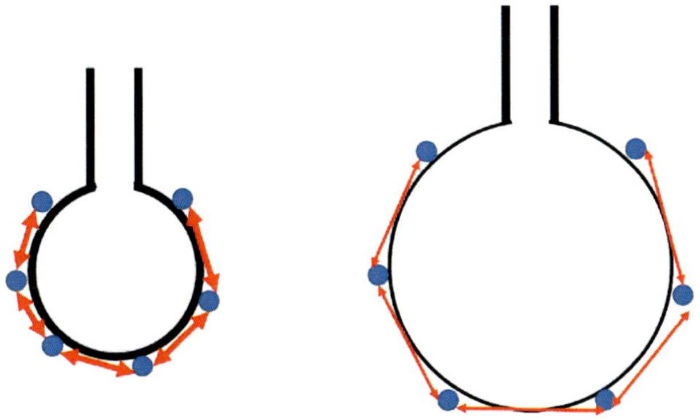

PEEP helps with this process by maintaining our progress along the way. As airway pressure increases on inhalation and the alveoli expand, PEEP essentially maintains that expansion on exhalation and prevents us from cycling back to that deflated, left-hand state in the above drawing. An added benefit of this is that it reduces stress on the alveoli. Going from deflated to inflated to deflated to inflated and on and on can damage the alveoli; PEEP decreases the difference between those two states so that less net movement is required for each inhalation. We talk about this more in the section on **Driving Pressure**, so no need for more detail at this point.

[87] Desai, 2012 – This video reviews the factors that determine the rate at which gasses diffuse across this membrane; we cite it again in the section on **Oxygenation** when we return to the idea

To summarize so far: PEEP is a residual pressure that we leave in the alveoli during exhalation to both maximize pulmonary respiration and maintain recruitment of alveoli.[88] So now that we have that clarified, let's look at a waveform representing pressure into the system as we deliver a breath. We've seen this image previously, but now we are going to add to it. The first breath is with no PEEP or zero PEEP or "ZEEP," the second one (right) is with 5cmH$_2$0 worth of PEEP added in:

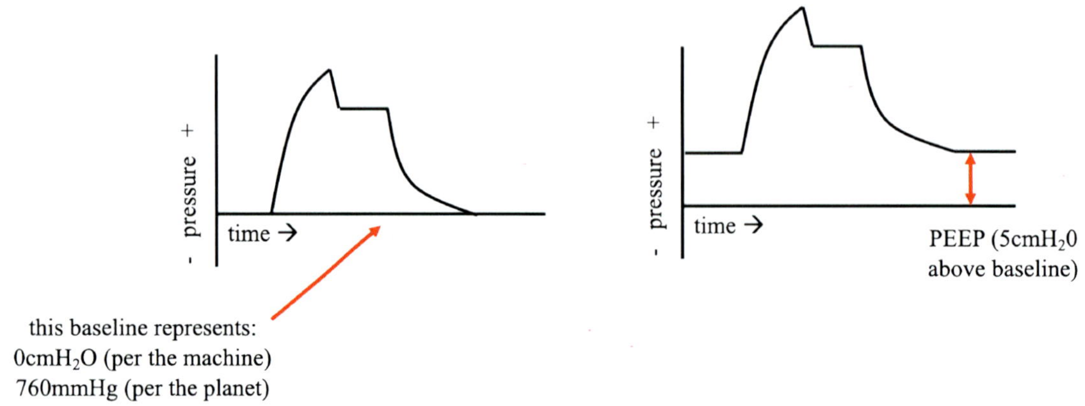

And to visualize this same idea over time, let's think of it this way:

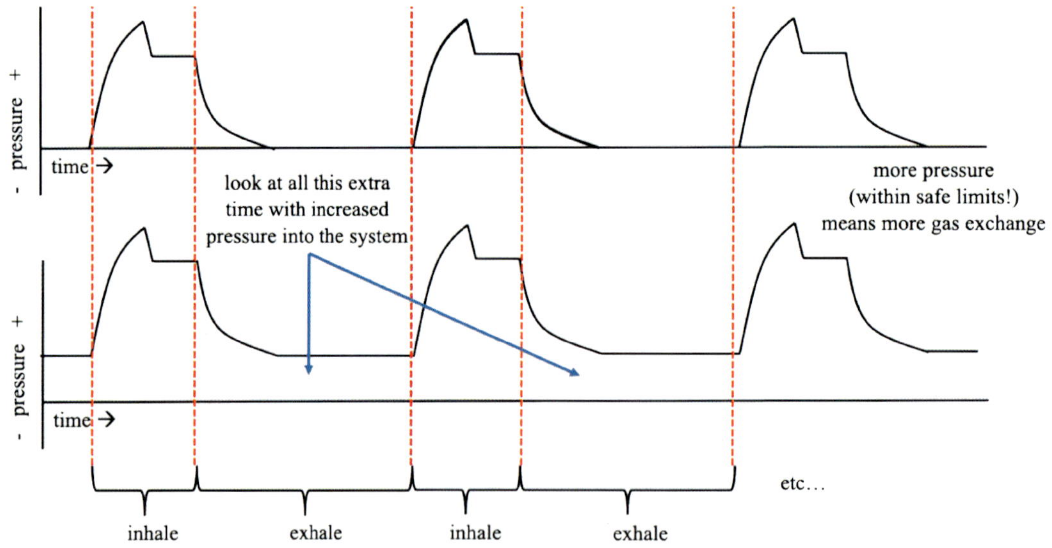

[88] Kallet & Branson, 2016 – While the focus of this article is on oxygen delivery (and we cite it later in **Oxygenation**), they also explain that PEEP doesn't necessarily open the alveoli as we often hear it described, rather PEEP keeps the alveoli open after inspiratory pressure changes (or **Recruitment Maneuvers**) open them up; also, to review the idea of pulmonary respiration look back to the section on **Terms to Describe Breathing**

MV – minute volume; **OK** – alright; **PALS** – pediatric advanced life support; **PEEP** – positive end-expiratory pressure; **PSI** – pounds per square inch; **RR** – respiratory rate; **s** – second; **TV** – tidal volume

Now this is not to say that gas exchange is nonexistent on exhalation in the first (no PEEP) case, just that it is augmented during the second one. There are also other mechanisms by which PEEP facilitates **Oxygenation**, but those will come up shortly. The important thing to note for now is that PEEP acts to keep alveoli open during exhalation and that helps us utilize more lung volume while breathing for the patient.

Let's next take a look at the downsides of PEEP. The most relevant one to mention is that PEEP can decrease cardiac output.[89] Recall from a previous discussion that any increase in intrathoracic pressure can impede blood flow back to the heart. Because of this, normal PEEP is less than 10cmH$_2$0. That said, we sometimes use PEEP up to 20cmH$_2$0 in specific cases and we will talk about those later. Other negative consequences of PEEP vary widely from things like worsening hypoxia and increased ventilation/ perfusion (V/Q) mismatch to decreased extra-thoracic organ function and decreased cerebral perfusion pressure.[90] That said, the important thing is that these negative effects typically manifest when the application of PEEP is taken beyond the level of therapeutic benefit. To phrase it a different way: use PEEP when needed, but don't assume it is without consequences, and be sure to utilize it judiciously. And the specifics for how we go about that will be discussed shortly.

---

[89] Clinical Analysis Management, 2009; Strong, 2013 – This effect of decreased cardiac output due to PEEP isn't so much a thing with a well-hydrated patient, so we can mitigate that somewhat by giving fluids if our patient will tolerate it

[90] Coruh & Luks, 2014; Luecke & Pelosi, 2005 – Refer to these sources for detailed explanations of all of those negative consequences of PEEP

cmH₂O – centimeters of water; **FiO₂** – fraction of inspired oxygen; **IBW** – ideal body weight; **I:E** – inspiratory to expiratory; **I-time** – inspiratory time; **kg** – kilogram; **LPM** – liters per minute; **min** – minute; **ml** – milliliter; **mmHg** – millimeters of mercury

Inspiratory Time (and I:E Ratio)

The next term to consider is inspiratory time (I-time), which is the amount of time over which we deliver a breath. It varies by age as so:[91]

age description	age (years)	I-time (s)
infant	.083 (1 month) – 1	0.3 – 0.7
toddler	1 – 2	0.4 – 0.9
preschooler	3 – 5	0.5 – 0.9
school-aged child	6 – 7	0.6 – 1.1
big kid	8 – 9	0.6 – 1.2
preadolescent	10 – 12	0.7 – 1.4
adolescent	12 – 15	0.8 – 1.7
adult	16 and up	0.8 – 1.7

One idea related to positive-pressure ventilation is that the more time we spend pushing air into system, the more oxygen gets moved into the bloodstream. This means that more time spent on the inspiration side of the breath cycle (versus exhalation) equals better **Oxygenation**.[92] With that in mind, one way to increase time spent at inspiration would be to lengthen the inspiratory time. If we do that, however, we have to accommodate by decreasing time spent at expiration or by decreasing **Respiratory Rate**. Consider seventeen breaths over one minute:

$$60\text{s} \div 17 \text{ breaths} \approx 3.5\text{s per breath}$$

$$\text{if in or inspiration} = 1.0\text{s},$$
$$\text{then out or exhalation} = 3.5\text{s} - 1.0\text{s}$$
$$\text{out or exhalation} = 2.5\text{s}$$

$$\text{if we lengthen inspiratory time to } 1.5\text{s:}$$
$$\text{exhalation time} = 3.5\text{s} - 1.5\text{s}$$
$$= 2.0\text{s}$$

[91] See **Appendix** for how we got all these values for normal inspiratory times based on age

[92] This idea of utilizing inspiratory time to facilitate oxygenation is also discussed when we get to **Mean Airway Pressure**

We often represent this ratio between inspiratory time and expiratory time as an I:E ratio to describe the amount of time spent at inspiration in comparison to the amount of time spent at exhalation. A normal I:E ratio is anywhere from 1:2 – 1:3.[93] Let's build an I:E ratio for the above examples:

in the first example, we have 1.0s : 2.5s, so our I:E ratio is 1:2.5

in the second example, we lengthened our inspiratory time to 1.5s;
so we now have 1.5s : 2.0s

now we need to simplify the ratio so that one of the numbers is 1:
simply divide both sides by the smaller number: $\frac{1.5}{1.5}:\frac{2.0}{1.5}$
and solve for our new I:E ratio of 1:1.33

To bring it back home: we had a rate of 17 and an inspiratory time of 1.0s with a resultant I:E ratio of 1:2.5. We wanted to increase time spent at inspiration, so we changed our inspiratory time to 1.5s and ended up with an I:E ratio of 1:1.33. For now we don't have to worry about the significance of these numbers, we just need to understand the math, how we get to these numbers, and the terminology associated with them. Let's try another example, but this time we will adjust rate instead of inspiratory time:

per above: RR of 17, I-time 1.0s = I:E ratio of 1:2.5
now let's increase our rate to 20 and recalculate the I:E ratio
60s ÷ 20 breaths = 3s per breath

if in or inspiration = 1.0s, then out or exhalation = 3.0s – 1.0s
therefore out or exhalation = 2.0s

in this example, we now have 1.0s : 2.0s, so our I:E ratio is 1:2.0

now let's shorten our I-time to 0.8s and see what happens:
if in or inspiration = 0.8s, then out or exhalation = 3.0s – 0.8s
therefore out or exhalation = 2.2s

now we have 0.8s : 2.2s,
but we need to make this an I:E ratio with a value of 1:
$\frac{0.8}{0.8}:\frac{2.2}{0.8} = 1:2.75$

[93] Yartsev, 2019 - To clarify this idea: a normal I:E ratio for the spontaneously breathing patient is in the neighborhood of 1:2, but often times we see something more like 1:3 with vented patients because we leave inspiratory time alone at a default of 1.0s – because of this convention and the facts that it is both common practice and generally well-tolerated, we've stated things as we did and will carry on with this assumption

cmH₂O – centimeters of water; **FiO₂** – fraction of inspired oxygen; **IBW** – ideal body weight; **I:E** – inspiratory to expiratory; **I-time** – inspiratory time; **kg** – kilogram; **LPM** – liters per minute; **min** – minute; **ml** – milliliter; **mmHg** – millimeters of mercury

Last thing to touch on is how we describe these different I:E ratios. To make sense of this, consider the I:E ratios as fractions or decimal numbers:

$$1{:}1 = \frac{1}{1} = 1$$

$$1{:}2 = \frac{1}{2} = 0.5$$

$$1{:}4 = \frac{1}{4} = 0.25$$

In this sense, an I:E ratio of 1:2 can be decreased to 1:4 or increased to 1:1. We can decrease I:E ratio by either decreasing inspiratory time or decreasing rate. Likewise, we can increase the I:E ratio via a longer inspiratory time or higher respiratory rate. We can also describe an I:E ratio with terms such as lengthen, extend, and prolong to describe change in one direction or shorten to describe changes in the opposite direction. Just know that there isn't an accepted convention with this terminology, so to say "lengthen or extend an I:E ratio" is a bit ambiguous and could describe a change in either direction. That said, it is probably better to simply describe the expiratory time itself or to outline a specific action taken:

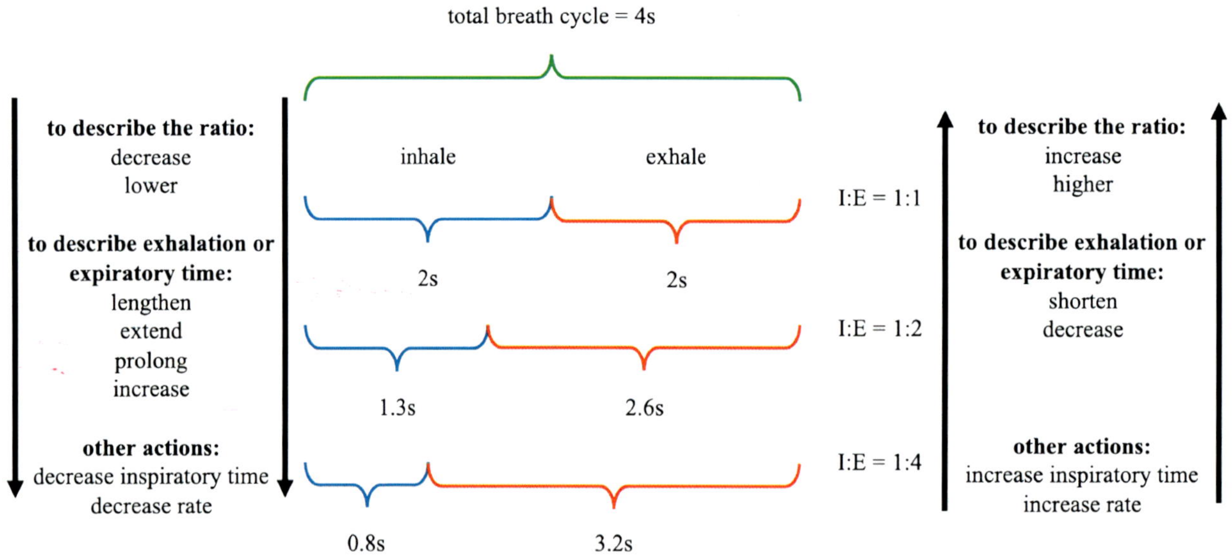

MV – minute volume; **OK** – alright; **PALS** – pediatric advanced life support; **PEEP** – positive end-expiratory pressure; **PSI** – pounds per square inch; **RR** – respiratory rate; **s** – second; **TV** – tidal volume

One final point here is that some machines allow us to select an I:E ratio directly and then inspiratory time is calculated automatically based on the chosen ratio and respiratory rate. While it is more common that inspiratory time is the independent variable and I:E ratio is calculated based on that, as we've just outlined things, both options do exist.

Let's summarize this all one more time and make a few generalizations: we can increase our I:E ratio by either increasing inspiratory time or increasing rate; we can decrease our I:E ratio by decreasing inspiratory time or decreasing rate. A higher I:E ratio means less time (in relation to the whole in/out cycle) spent on exhalation, a smaller or lower I:E ratio means more time for exhalation. We will talk about this later when we get to ventilator strategies, but know that some patients can benefit from a shorter I:E ratio and other can benefit from a longer I:E ratio, so it is important to know which changes affect the I:E ratio in which direction.

ARDS – acute respiratory distress syndrome; **cmH_2O** – centimeters of water; **COPD** – chronic obstructive pulmonary disease

Types of Breaths

Let's take a few minutes to discuss an image we presented towards the beginning of this manual. We want to explain in a little more detail each of the following types of breaths depicted below:[94]

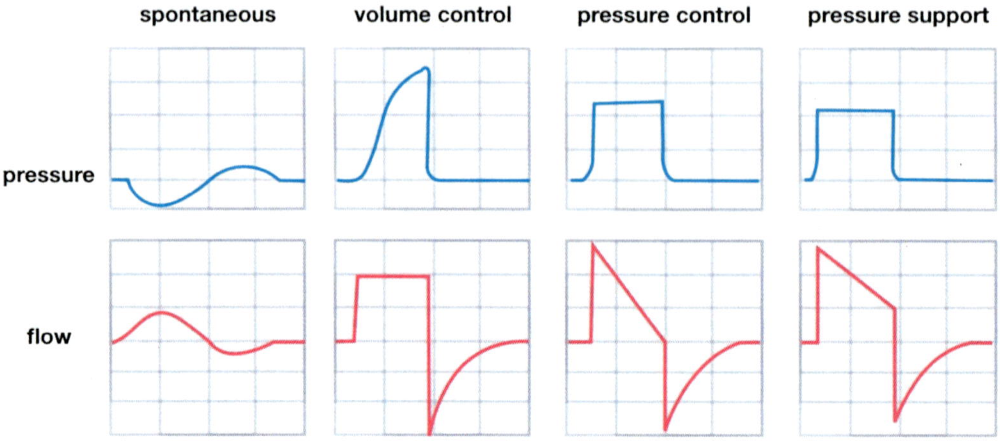

There are two waveforms depicted for each type of breath, pressure and flow, each shown over time. We sometimes hear these graphics of vent function described as scalars, as in a pressure-time scalar or flow-time scalar.[95] The image above shows ideal scalar waveforms, real ones as produced by a vent may vary somewhat and will be less clean-cut than these guys. But enough on that for now, let's move on to each of these things: pressure and flow.

---

[94] We mentioned it already, but this graphic was built by Dr. Sameer of *Art by Dr. Sam* on Fiverr and *The Young Orthopod* on YouTube

[95] Iyer & Holets, 2016 – Since we don't typically have access to waveforms in transport, we'll defer a discussion of it here; that said, refer to this presentation for a brief overview

I:E – inspiratory to expiratory; **OK** – alright; **PEEP** – positive end-expiratory pressure; **s** – second; **SIMV** – synchronized intermittent mandatory ventilation

Pressure is measured by the machine somewhere between the endotracheal tube and the wye where the inhalation side of the circuit splits off from the exhalation side of the circuit:[96]

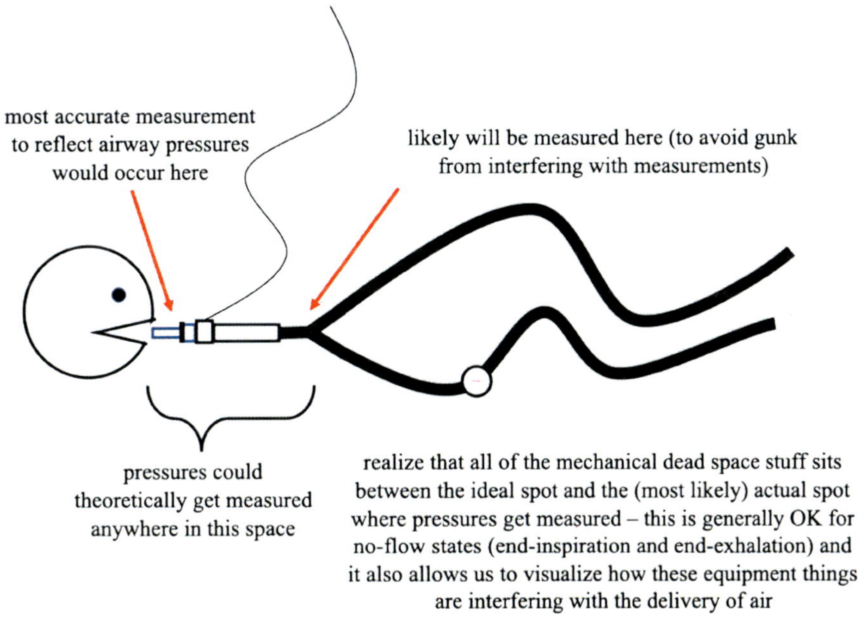

Another thing to mention is that the pressures we measure don't directly describe pressures at the alveoli or terminal ends of the airway, they reflect what's going on outside of the patient's body. That said, we can manipulate the system to approximate alveolar pressures (and we will discuss how to do that later) and we assume that the value we measure correlates with average pressure at the alveoli. Pressures experienced by individual alveoli vary throughout the lung and our measurement occurs outside of the lungs themselves, but this is the best we have and therefore we base our treatment on the information available to us. The waveform that shows pressure over time gives us a visual representation of how pressure changes at the mouth side of the system as we deliver a breath. And we already talked about how pressure is measured (in terms of units), so we are good on this general idea for now.

[96] Hess, 2014 – We'll cite this article a few more times, it provides alternative explanations for many of the things we'll discuss along the way; specific to this section, however, it briefly describes where within the circuit pressures can be measured

ARDS – acute respiratory distress syndrome; **cmH_2O** – centimeters of water; **COPD** – chronic obstructive pulmonary disease

Next concept to discuss is flow. Flow is a description of how fast we move air through the system and is quantified in liters per minute (LPM).[97] When we describe flow, we do so at the machine side of the system. As air moves away from the machine, however, different things can interfere with the speed at which the body of air is moving. We create flow and send it to the patient via the machine, then we see all of this interference indirectly via other parameters (such as pressures and volumes). Here's how it looks mapped out on top of the system:

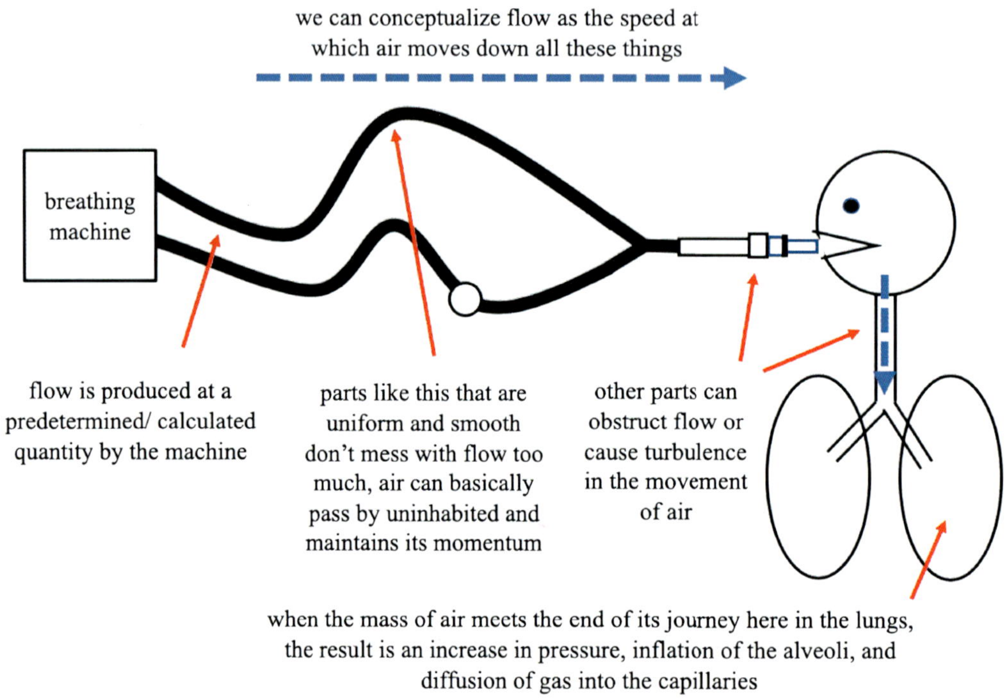

[97] And sometimes flow is notated by the symbol $\dot{V}$, but we also use that same symbol in Fick's Law stuff in the next section and don't want to get things confused…

I:E – inspiratory to expiratory; **OK** – alright; **PEEP** – positive end-expiratory pressure; **s** – second; **SIMV** – synchronized intermittent mandatory ventilation

Now that we are set on the basics of pressure (as measured in the system) and flow (as produced by the machine), let's look at a few of these waveforms again and see how we can deliver breaths in different ways:

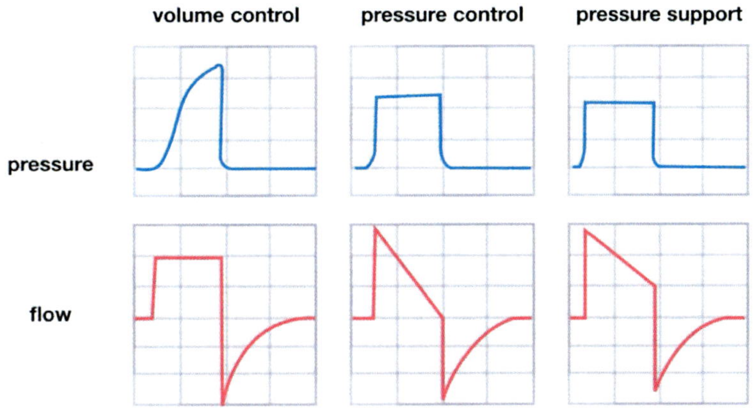

The first thing to note is that there are three general categories: volume control breaths, pressure control breaths, and pressure support breaths.[98] In volume control, a breath is most commonly delivered via a square-waveform flow pattern in which the machine spins up to a set flow, holds it for a predetermined amount of time, then cycles off. With pressure control and pressure support breaths, however, flow is delivered via a decelerating-waveform flow pattern in which the machine starts a breath by spinning up to a max pressure and then slowly maintaining that pressure by delivering decreasing flow until the breath cycles off. To say this all another way: volume control gives constant flow for variable pressure, pressure control and pressure support give constant pressure at variable flow.

Let's follow this up with a series of sequential facts: There are some machines nowadays that can give volume control breaths via a decelerating flow pattern, but those aren't available in the transport setting.[99] That means we can lump these three types of breaths into two groups: volume/ constant flow and pressure/ decelerating flow. Unless we are in volume control and SIMV, we ventilate patients with one type of breath at a time. In very general terms: the pressure/ decelerating-waveform breaths are more comfortable for patients but take longer to deliver (i.e. may not be ideal when we need to give breaths fast or allow lots of time for exhalation).[100]

---

[98] And recognize that breaths delivered in **Pressure-Regulated Volume Control** fall into the **Pressure Control** category

[99] Gonzales & friends, 2012 – At least we are pretty sure the option of decelerating flow in volume control doesn't exist in any transport ventilators, but new products come up all the time; amongst many other fun things, the article explains how pressure/ decelerating-waveform breaths may be best for ARDS patients and volume/ square-waveform breaths may be best for obstruction related to COPD

[100] Iyer & Holets, 2016 – And in this presentation on vent waveforms, they describe how longer inspiratory times may be indicated for patients vented with a decelerating-waveform pattern

ARDS – acute respiratory distress syndrome; **cmH₂O** – centimeters of water; **COPD** – chronic obstructive pulmonary disease

As for the two types of pressure/ decelerating-pattern breaths (pressure control and pressure support), there are a few things to mention. First is that the pressure used to describe these breaths can either be referred to in addition to PEEP or inclusive of PEEP. We describe the value as cumulative or absolute to include PEEP or additive to say it is added on top of PEEP.[101] This varies by machine, so just be aware of it:

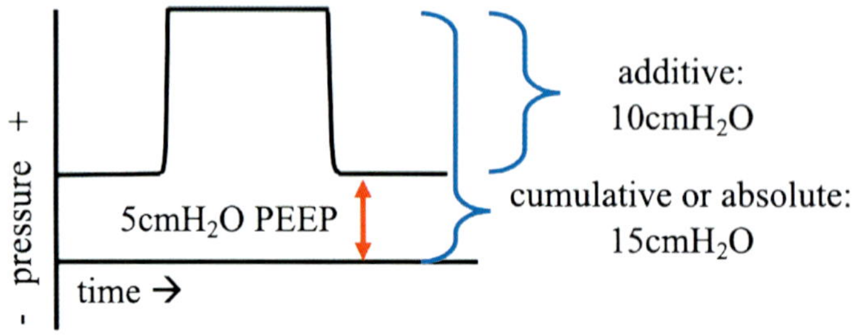

Another concept to discuss is rise time. This term describes how fast we get from zero to our set inspiratory pressure (either in pressure control or with a pressure support breath). Different machines describe and label this parameter differently, but the general idea is that a shorter rise time means the pressure gets up to what we have set more quickly.[102] This isn't something we mess around with too often in transport, but it is good to know if we are troubleshooting issues. Just keep in mind that a higher or longer rise time may mean less tidal volume if inspiratory time is not adjusted (i.e. lengthened) to accommodate that change. And then if inspiratory time changes, we may end up with less time for expiration (i.e. we will have an increased or larger I:E ratio). Again, not something we routinely mess with in invasive ventilation, but it is good to know.

[101] Ashworth & friends, 2018, Bauer, 2016a – The first mentions this idea of describing pressure control or pressure support relative to PEEP in the context of pressure control ventilation; the second reviews this idea as it relates to non-invasive positive-pressure ventilation (which we don't get into here in this manual)
[102] Yartsev, 2019 – For a more detailed discussion of rise time and how things differ between machines, navigate here

I:E – inspiratory to expiratory; **OK** – alright; **PEEP** – positive end-expiratory pressure; **s** – second; **SIMV** – synchronized intermittent mandatory ventilation

The next thing to mention here is how pressure control and pressure support breaths differ. While both are given via a decelerating-waveform pattern, the mechanism by which the breath cycles off changes things. A pressure control breath is designed to deliver a full breath even with no patient effort, whereas a pressure support breath is designed to simply relieve some effort of breathing on the front end of a breath. Because of this difference, a comparable titration of pressure (i.e. a change of 5cmH_2O for both pressure control and pressure support) may result in different changes of volume in the very same patient. Now the mechanism by which this works is known as termination, the parameter by which the machine decides to stop supporting a breath and begin exhalation:[103]

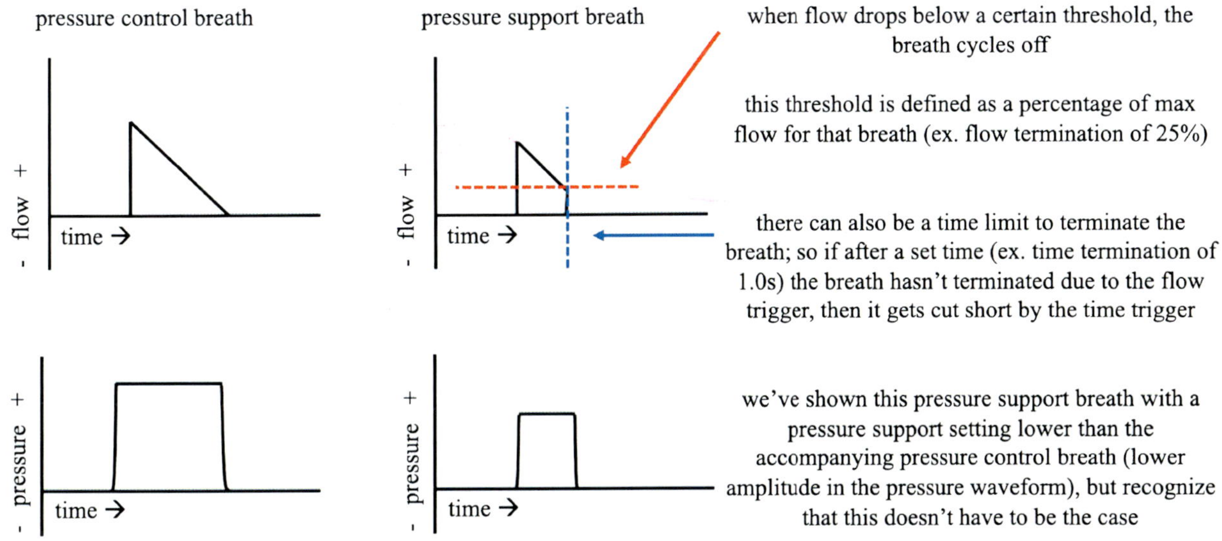

So to get more volume in a pressure support breath (represented by the area under the flow-time waveform), we either need more patient effort (i.e. don't take away a patient's respiratory drive with too much sedation) or we need to maximize our termination triggers (i.e. lower value for flow termination, longer time termination).[104] We don't typically get that far into the weeds with invasive ventilation and pressure support, but we will often see this idea discussed in terms of non-invasive ventilation (which, again, we don't cover in this manual).

[103] To expand on this, the term cycle refers to how the machine decides to stop giving a breath in a general sense, termination as we've drawn it out is specific to pressures support breaths

[104] The primary mechanism for terminating a pressures support breath will be the flow termination and it may help to think of the time termination as a backup in the event that the breath doesn't end via the flow termination mechanism

ARDS – acute respiratory distress syndrome; **cmH₂O** – centimeters of water; **COPD** – chronic obstructive pulmonary disease

Last bit of this section: let's review different types of breaths as they relate to time-triggered, patient-triggered, assisted, supported, and unassisted (which is slightly different than they were described in that first image in the section). We touched on these as we moved through the different modes, but we'll just clarify a few things and show how they vary from one to another starting with a graphic:

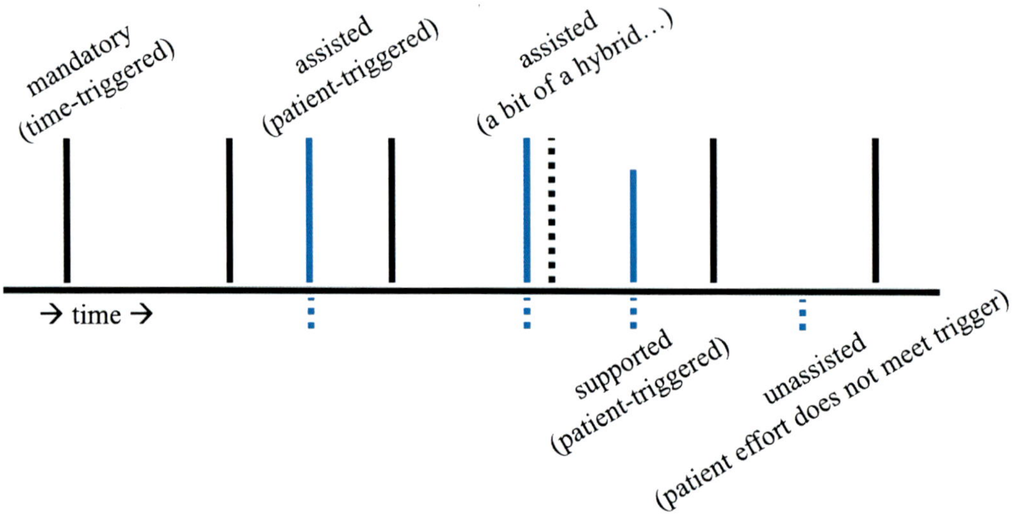

Mandatory or time-triggered breaths are the ones that we deliver via our set rate on the vent and to a specific goal, whether that be volume or pressure. Assisted breaths are triggered by patient effort and then the machine delivers a full breath to match the same goal as for the machine-delivered ones.[105] Moving right, supported breaths are also patient-triggered, but get delivered via pressure support and not to a set goal. Supported breaths are often smaller than mandatory or assisted ones (in terms of volume), that's why they have been shown with a shorter blue line.[106] And lastly is spontaneous effort that doesn't get supported or assisted - these efforts get ignored by the machine and function solely via patient effort.

[105] Chatburn & friends, 2014 – For more on that hybrid situation, take a look here; these guys would identify it as a machine-triggered breath, but since we started our discussion with a differentiation between time- and patient-triggers we will just refer you to their article – the labeling doesn't change our treatment

[106] But again, this doesn't necessarily have to be the case and we can, in fact, work to have pressure support breaths equal in volume to those mandatory or time-triggered ones; see section on **Synchronized Intermittent Mandatory Ventilation** for more on this

I:E – inspiratory to expiratory; **OK** – alright; **PEEP** – positive end-expiratory pressure; **s** – second; **SIMV** – synchronized intermittent mandatory ventilation

To take this discussion one step further, let's consider which types of breaths apply to which types of ventilation. In assist control we have time-triggered or mandatory breaths and assisted breaths. In SIMV we have time-triggered or mandatory breaths, assisted breaths (when a trigger is sensed within the mandatory period), and supported breaths (when a trigger is sensed in the spontaneous period). In neither mode do we see spontaneous effort that meets the trigger threshold and does not get assisted in some way. While there may be spontaneous effort that doesn't meet the trigger (and this theoretically could contribute some to minute volume), all noteworthy patient effort (defined by meeting whatever trigger threshold we have set) will get facilitated by the machine in some way in either mode.[107]

[107] And we realize that we've talked a lot about **Triggers** here, but the details on that have been deferred until later on

ARDS – acute respiratory distress syndrome; **cmH_2O** – centimeters of water; **FiO_2** – fraction of inspired oxygen; **Hgb** – hemoglobin; **I:E** – inspiratory to expiratory; **mmHg** – millimeters of mercury; **O_2** – oxygen

Three Big Things

There are three very important things that need to be monitored and addressed for all ventilated patients, hands down and no matter what. The order in which we discuss them here is totally arbitrary as they all hold equal weight and are interrelated. The ideas that follow are in general terms and not specific to certain pathologies or patient types. All those details will come later.

Oxygenation

It may have come up once or twice before, but oxygen is pretty important stuff. Oxygen gets to tissues via a few steps, some of those we can affect directly with the ventilator. Let's start with a version of a graphic we used earlier that shows partial pressures at a few steps along the way in the spontaneously breathing patient:[108]

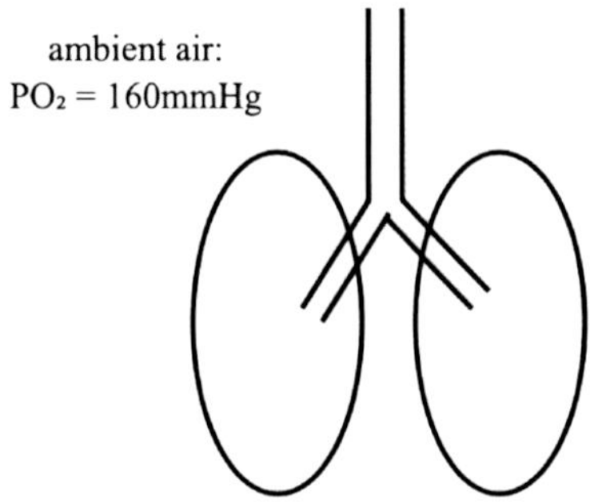

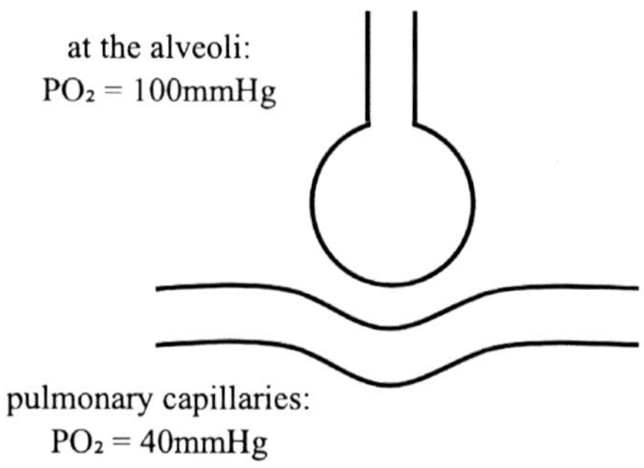

[108] Bauer, 2016c – Take a look at this short article for a review of Henry's Law and the concept of PO_2 at the pulmonary capillaries, offers a preview of how we can improve oxygenation in the ventilated patient (the steps of which we will lay out in this section)

OK – alright; **PaO_2** – partial pressure of arterial oxygen; **PEEP** – positive end-expiratory pressure; **PO_2** – partial pressure of oxygen; **PvO_2** – partial pressure of venous oxygen; **SpO_2** – pulse oximetry

Recognize that gasses will diffuse from areas of high concentration to areas of lower concentration. In this baseline example, oxygen will move from the ambient air to the alveoli, then into the pulmonary capillaries. The first way that we can speed this process up is by changing the partial pressure of oxygen at the start of the system. Instead of 21% of the gas mix or 160mmHg of oxygen, we can titrate that all the way up to 100% (**Fraction of Inspired Oxygen** 1.0) or 760mmHg. This will increase the rate at which oxygen diffuses to the alveoli, resulting in a higher partial pressure of oxygen downstream and, subsequently, faster diffusion into the bloodstream:

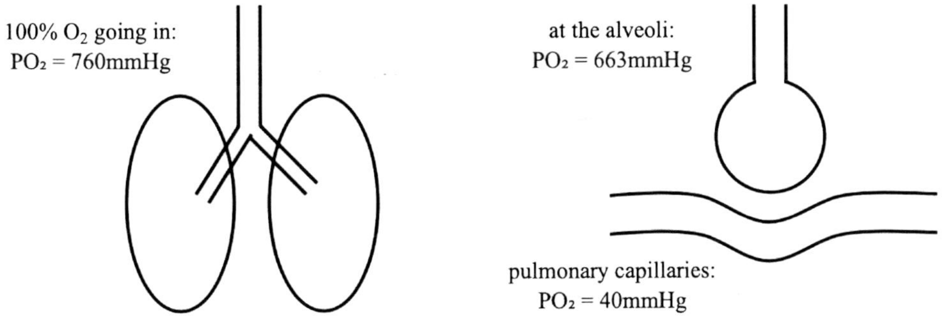

Let's recap this bit and do some math: PO_2 at the alveoli on ambient air is 160mmHg, PO_2 at 100% FiO_2 is 663mmHg. To quantify the result of this difference let's apply Fick's Law:[109]

$$\dot{V} = \frac{(P_1 - P_2) \text{ x area x D}}{\text{thickness}}$$

$\dot{V}$ = rate of gas diffusion across a membrane (i.e. at the alveolar membrane)

P_1 = ingoing pressure (i.e. to the alveoli)

P_2 = pressure at other side (i.e. in the blood)

area = self-explanatory…

D = diffusion constant for a particular gas (oxygen in this case)

thickness = also self-explanatory…

if $\frac{\text{area x D}}{\text{thickness}}$ is constant and we call it k,

we end up with the following:

$$\dot{V} = (P_1 - P_2)k$$

[109] Desai, 2012 – This video, courtesy of Khan Academy, outlines all of these factors with an animated depiction of Fick's Law

and let's add in some numbers for the ambient air and 100% FiO_2 situations:

$$\dot{V}_{\text{ambient air}} = (100 - 40)k$$
$$= 60k$$

$$\dot{V}_{100\%\ \text{oxygen}} = (663 - 40)k$$
$$= 623k$$

That means that oxygen diffusion occurs ten times faster at 100% (or a FiO_2 of 1.0) than at room air. Which is both nuts and a clinically significant thing to be aware of. The takeaway here is that whenever we need to increase the diffusion of gas across the alveolar membrane, FiO_2 is a heck of a way to get that done. The holdup is when other factors in the equation (area and thickness) are also issues or if the problem is with oxygen transport after the point at which it diffuses into the blood. In those cases we may need to augment this strategy with other techniques, as we will discuss real soon.[110]

Another thing to mention here is that oxygen can cause damage when given in excess of physiologic need for a sustained amount of time. Now the timeline at which the stuff can occur is likely longer than our transport, but that doesn't mean we need to get reckless and ventilate everyone with an FiO_2 of 100%. We'll talk in just a moment about how we evaluate oxygenation and the idea is to make sure a need is met while being conscious that all interventions, even something as seemingly benign as oxygen, have consequences.[111]

To expand on this idea just a bit before we move on, one specific argument against a high FiO_2 is the idea of absorption atelectasis – the closing of alveoli related to nitrogen washout and the fact that oxygen quickly diffuses into the bloodstream leaving less gas in the alveoli.[112] While the clinical impact of this sequence of events is up for debate and may not actually make a difference, it is something that comes up in the discussion of vented patients.[113] And if we do give credence to the idea, ways to mitigate this effect would be maintaining a patient's spontaneous effort to breath (discussed shortly in **Comfort**) and performing **Recruitment Maneuvers** (discussed much later).[114]

---

[110] Murphy, 2017b; Macintyre, 2014 – And to review the different types of hypoxia, take a look at this video (lots of detail, reviews the four types as we often label them in critical care transport) and that article (different system of considering the various causes, but equally informative)

[111] Kallet & Branson, 2016 – This article looks at both why it may make sense to limit oxygenation and how the negative consequences of oxygen may be exaggerated

[112] Dunphy, 2012 – Short video that explains both the mechanism of absorption atelectasis and how patient effort can mitigate the effect

[113] Yartsev, 2019 – This article both sheds some doubt on the idea of absorption atelectasis and describes many of the other mechanisms by which oxygen can adversely affect our patients

[114] Hartland & friends, 2015; Radermacher & friends, 2017 - The first article outlines an argument for the use of recruitment maneuvers in certain patients (which seems reasonable to extrapolate to some of the patients we see in the transport setting); the second specifically addresses this idea that recruitment maneuvers are of benefit with absorption atelectasis

OK – alright; **PaO_2** – partial pressure of arterial oxygen; **PEEP** – positive end-expiratory pressure; **PO_2** – partial pressure of oxygen; **PvO_2** – partial pressure of venous oxygen; **SpO_2** – pulse oximetry

Increasing FiO_2 is one way to get more oxygen into the bloodstream. While this isn't the fix for all types of hypoxia and there are some potential negatives, we generally start here when looking to address oxygenation issues. The next way we can increase oxygenation is via **Positive End-Expiratory Pressure**. Now PEEP doesn't quite work by the same mechanism, as the addition of PEEP doesn't much change the partial pressure situation as we saw with an increase in FiO_2:

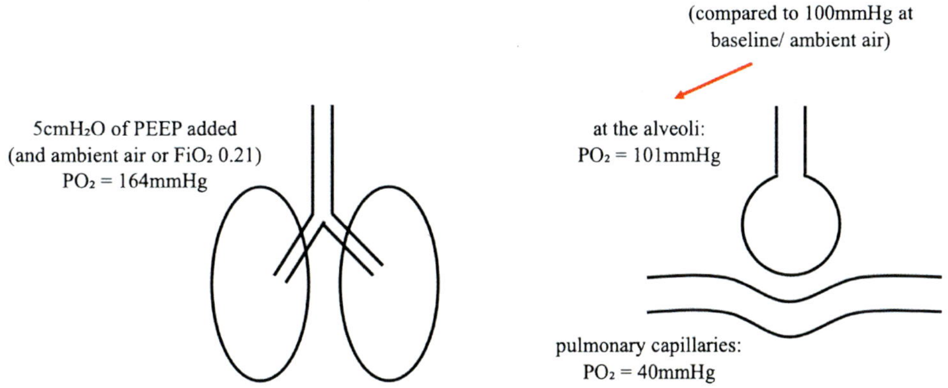

Instead, PEEP facilitates oxygenation primarily by increasing and thinning out the alveolar surface throughout the respiratory cycle. We discussed this concept way back in the section on **Alveolar Surface Area** and again just a moment ago in the section on **Positive End-Expiratory Pressure**, so no need to redo all of that here. One more mechanism by which PEEP helps oxygenation is that it cleans up the alveolar membrane, in a sense, by pushing out or displacing fluid that accumulates there. Think of it this way:

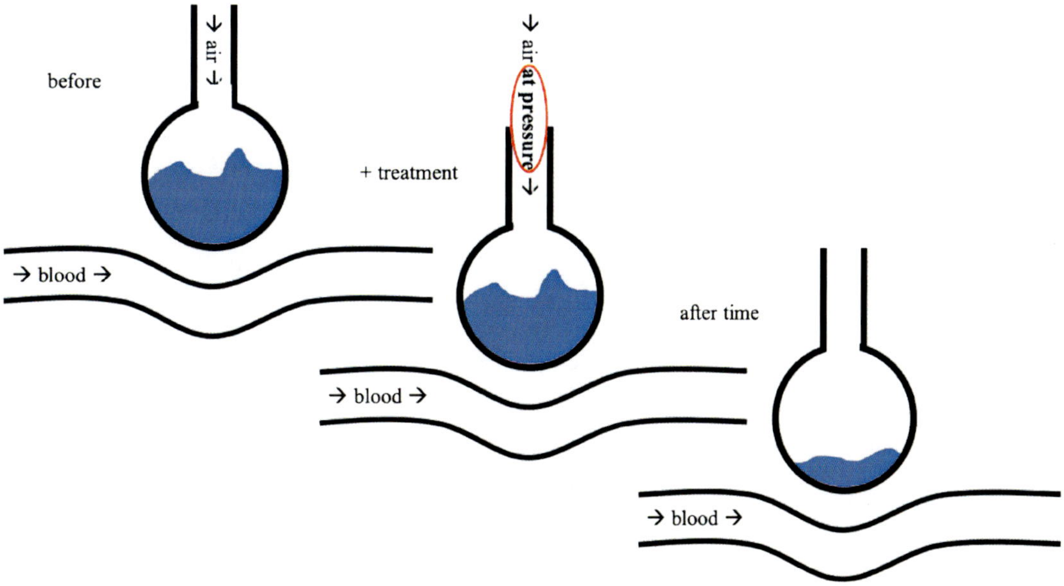

ARDS – acute respiratory distress syndrome; **cmH₂O** – centimeters of water; **FiO₂** – fraction of inspired oxygen; **Hgb** – hemoglobin; **I:E** – inspiratory to expiratory; **mmHg** – millimeters of mercury; **O₂** – oxygen

As a point of clarification on this idea, fluid in the alveoli doesn't necessarily impede gas exchange as much as we might think. As we mentioned before, carbon dioxide moves fairly efficiently through liquids.[115] Oxygenation, on the other hand, can be readily maintained by increasing PO_2 at the alveoli via both FiO_2 and PEEP as we just pointed out.[116] Edema in the alveoli (pulmonary edema) impairs oxygenation in roundabout ways. We'll mention these later, but one of the primary mechanisms of this is that edema makes alveoli more suspectable to damage in positive-pressure ventilation.[117] It also makes it harder for us to get air into the alveoli and increases work of breathing.[118] While fluid in the lungs does, in fact, impact the processes of oxygenation and ventilation, it's not exactly a straightforward diffusion problem.

But to get back on track with our discussion: assuming **Ventilation** and **Comfort** are adequate (see next sections), initial steps to fix oxygenation are increasing FiO_2 and then adding PEEP. While it's totally OK to use a stepwise approach that titrates both FiO_2 and PEEP in line with one another, recognize that FiO_2 is our most direct fix for improving partial pressure of oxygen at the alveoli and has few consequences in the acute (i.e. short term) setting.[119] PEEP, on the other hand, is especially helpful in facilitating gas exchange across the alveolar membrane and driving fluid out of the lungs, but may decrease cardiac output by way of a drop in preload to the heart (especially if our patient is down on fluids).[120] Lastly, both of these techniques (FiO_2 and PEEP) improve oxygenation throughout the respiratory cycle.

The next point to make is that all of the benefits of FiO_2 and PEEP (in the context of oxygenation) are further maximized during inspiration:

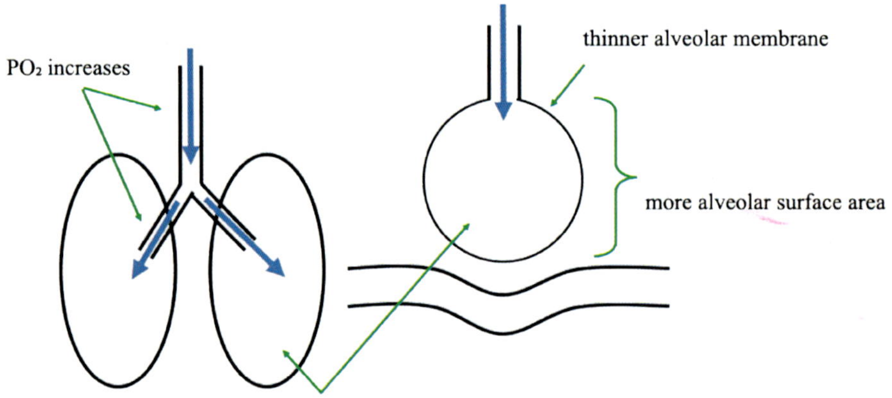

[115] Speller, 2018 – We first cited this article in **The Normal Breathing Process** when we talked about how both oxygen and carbon dioxide diffuse across the alveolar-capillary membrane
[116] Radermacher & friends, 2017 – This article discusses the management of ARDS (which we will get to later) and mentions this idea that the movement of gasses through liquid in the alveoli can be overcome relatively easily
[117] Perlman & friends, 2010 – Damage to the alveoli, whether from edema or any other cause, can lead to a cascade of effects that further impact both oxygenation and ventilation; this paper focuses on the specifics of how individual alveoli are affected by edema in neighboring alveoli
[118] Kuhn & friends, 2016 – We'll talk about **Compliance (and Resistance)** in a later section, but another way to say this is that edema decreases compliance
[119] We'll touch a bit more on this subject of titrating FiO_2 and PEEP together in the section on **Lung Injury**
[120] These negative consequences of positive-pressure ventilation were discussed in both **How is Positive-Pressure Ventilation Different?** and **Positive End-Expiratory Pressure**

OK – alright; **PaO_2** – partial pressure of arterial oxygen; **PEEP** – positive end-expiratory pressure; **PO_2** – partial pressure of oxygen; **PvO_2** – partial pressure of venous oxygen; **SpO_2** – pulse oximetry

This means that more time spent at inspiration further maximizes oxygenation, therefore strategy number three to improve oxygenation is to increase the **Inspiratory Time**. And changing inspiratory time consequently changes our I:E ratio. More specifically, increasing inspiratory time increases our I:E ratio (and shortens the expiratory time). For example, if we have an I:E ratio of 1:2 and then increase inspiratory time we might get an I:E ratio of 1:1. And then if we increase it enough, it will eventually become longer than exhalation and we end up with an inverted I:E ratio that might be written as 2:1. The primary drawback of a long inspiratory time (and of an inverted I:E ratio) is that it can be uncomfortable for our patients and we will need to get aggressive to maintain patient **Comfort**. An inverted I:E ratio may also make it tough for the patient to exhale fully, predisposing us to **AutoPEEP**.

Summary up to this point is that there are three ways to improve oxygenation by adjusting settings on the vent: increase FiO_2, add PEEP, and extend inspiratory time. Now why do we not just fill the lungs up with 100% oxygen and keep them inflated – we'd have a forever-long maximum diffusion of oxygen into the bloodstream, right? There are two reasons for this. One is that we don't want to affect hemodynamics indefinitely (as discussed above and previously). Two is that it isn't all about oxygen. We also have to consider its partner in crime, carbon dioxide, which doesn't diffuse so well in gas (as compared to oxygen) because it is a bigger, heavier molecule.[121] The movement of carbon dioxide, therefore, is partially dependent on the movement of the body of air in which it hangs out. And that leads us into our next section on **Ventilation**, but a few more things to cover before we get there.

Other things we can do to improve oxygenation include sitting our patient upright or elevating the head of bed,[122] ensuring adequate perfusion, utilizing more lung volume via **Recruitment Maneuvers**, and considering **Mean Airway Pressure**.[123] We won't get into the details of all of these things here, as the focus for now is on how to manipulate the machine.

[121] Flowers & friends, 2019 – This difference in how quickly oxygen and carbon dioxide move is explained by Graham's Law
[122] Spooner & friends, 2014 – While this article mainly focuses on lung volumes (which is a step or two removed from oxygenation), it goes into detail on the physiologic effects of elevating the vented patient's head
[123] While we could also make the argument that going up on respiratory rate increases the amount of time spent on inspiration, doing so also impacts ventilation (next section) so we generally don't consider rate one of the variables by which we control oxygenation

ARDS – acute respiratory distress syndrome; **cmH_2O** – centimeters of water; **FiO_2** – fraction of inspired oxygen; **Hgb** – hemoglobin; **I:E** – inspiratory to expiratory; **mmHg** – millimeters of mercury; **O_2** – oxygen

One more thing to consider is how we measure oxygenation. Our standard tool in the field is pulse oximetry or SpO_2. Pulse oximetry uses infrared to see to what extent our hemoglobin is saturated with oxygen (or oxygen-like things, but we won't worry about the tricky parts here).[124] The process goes like so: oxygen gets to the alveoli, it crosses into the bloodstream via diffusion gradients, then once in the bloodstream it gets picked up by hemoglobin for a ride down the blood vessel:

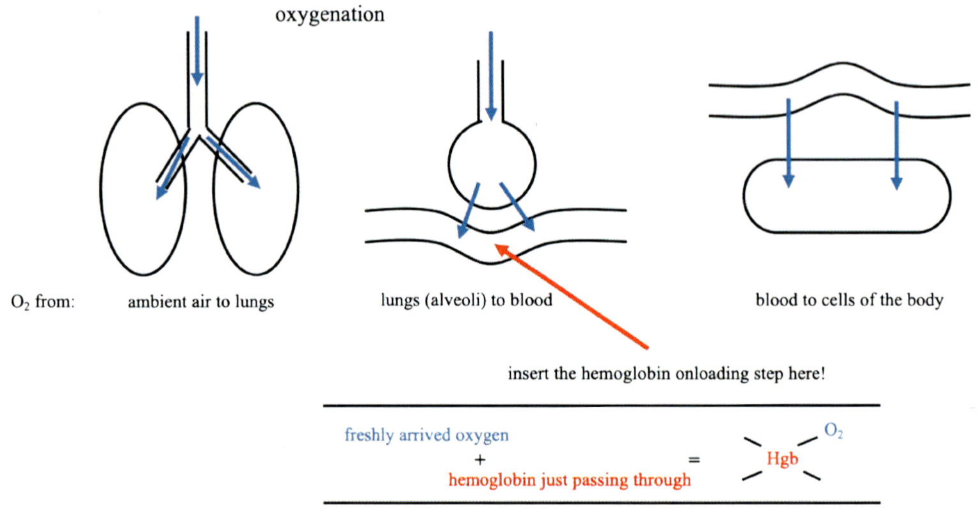

So we have a hemoglobin with four sites free, one of which is occupied by an oxygen molecule and the resultant hypothetical SpO_2 here is 25% (1 of 4 sites filled). Fill all four sites up and we are 100% saturated as so:

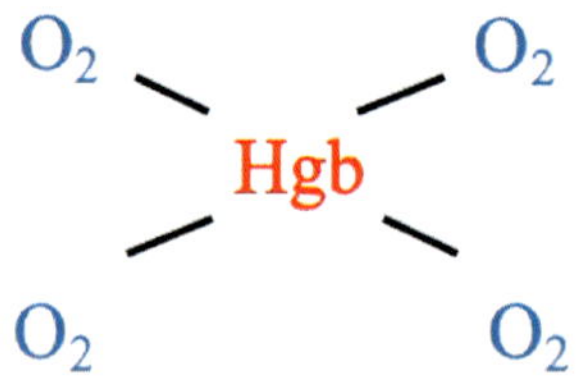

[124] Silverston, 2016 – Short article that describes both the technology and the limitations of pulse oximetry

OK – alright; **PaO_2** – partial pressure of arterial oxygen; **PEEP** – positive end-expiratory pressure; **PO_2** – partial pressure of oxygen; **PvO_2** – partial pressure of venous oxygen; **SpO_2** – pulse oximetry

Drawing it out this way is a bit of a simplification, but it does help us to understand what it is that pulse oximetry is looking at. Do note that hemoglobin doesn't cruise freely through the vessels, it comes attached to red blood cells (lots and lots of hemoglobin per each red blood cell), but the four sites per hemoglobin is a fair description. Also consider that we measure this saturation peripherally (hence the p in SpO_2). This means that if blood isn't getting to the periphery where we have our probe attached, numbers may not be accurate. And lastly, recall that as oxygen binds to that first site on the hemoglobin the physical shape of the hemoglobin molecule changes to attract subsequent oxygen molecules to the remaining vacant sites. This is why we aim for higher pulse oximetry values over 93% - once we get those hemoglobin molecules mostly filled up, it makes it way easier to fill up the remaining ones.

To carry on with this idea: when we get to 100% saturation, all further oxygen we put into the system will remain as dissolved oxygen in the blood. This has the potential to cause damage (as we've discussed before), so we tend to titrate pulse oximetry to an upper limit of 99%. We don't normally take our assessment of oxygenation much further than this in transport, but there are some programs that have the ability to measure blood gasses, so let's just touch on that for a moment. Partial pressure of arterial oxygen (PaO_2) allows us to see how much oxygen is dissolved in the bloodstream on the arterial side of the circulatory system. If we have an SpO_2 of 100% and a normal PaO_2, then our potential for causing damage is less than if we had a saturation of 100% and a markedly elevated PaO_2.

There are, however, many things that impact this relationship. Different factors can change hemoglobin's affinity for oxygen (and carbon dioxide) and we can better understand values for SpO_2 and its relationship to PaO_2 by considering this affect. For example, we may see a low SpO_2 paired with a normal PaO_2 to indicate that hemoglobin isn't holding on to oxygen as well as normal. This gets a bit beyond the scope of our discussion, but we'll return back to this idea later on when we talk about **Acidosis** to give some concrete examples and clinical application.[125] Just keep in mind that PaO_2 provide as snapshot in time, while pulse oximetry provides a continuous stream of information.[126]

One very last thing about this and then we'll get on to other things. There is some potential for utilizing partial pressure of venous oxygen (PvO_2) in the transport setting. PvO_2 samples are normally mixed-venous samples from a central line, but we could measure the partial pressure of oxygen from any blood source, to include venous blood from a normal venipuncture. Now blood on the venous side has already passed the capillary beds and therefore is dependent on delivery, metabolic need at the tissues, and offloading, so we would need to keep those things in mind. And in fact, there have been investigations into how we could use a peripheral blood gas to direct treatment if we do keep these other components in mind.[127] It's not that common at this point, but neither are arterial sticks in transport; using a PvO_2 could be a bridge to fill that gap.

[125] Hasudungan, 2018 – To dig more into this idea of what can affect hemoglobin's affinity for oxygen, refer to this video (and it also applies to the following section)
[126] Farkas, 2016 – This piece outlines a number of situations in which pulse oximetry might be preferred to the arterial blood gas
[127] Chemtob & Moller-Sorenson, 2018 – These guys looked into this concept of utilizing a PvO_2 with a peripheral venous sample to direct and guide treatment

ARDS – acute respiratory distress syndrome; **cmH_2O** – centimeters of water; **FiO_2** – fraction of inspired oxygen; **Hgb** – hemoglobin; **I:E** – inspiratory to expiratory; **mmHg** – millimeters of mercury; **O_2** – oxygen

One last summary before moving on from oxygenation. Oxygenation is one of the three big things in mechanical ventilation. We measure it via pulse oximetry, which tells us how filled up with oxygen the hemoglobin molecules (attached to red blood cells) in the blood are as they move past wherever we have attached the pulse oximetry probe. To get a better number (or improve oxygenation) by moving things around on the vent interface, we have three options and we typically do them in this order: increase FiO_2, add PEEP, and lengthen inspiratory tine. All that said, let's not forget the basics: position the patient appropriately, verify that perfusion is adequate, and make sure ventilation and comfort are addressed simultaneously (see next sections).[128]

[128] And to link to these other ideas: **Fraction of Inspired Oxygen, Positive End-Expiratory Pressure, Inspiratory Time (and I:E Ratio)**; **Ventilation, Comfort**

MV – minute volume; **O_2** – oxygen; **PEEP** – positive end-expiratory pressure; **VA** – alveolar minute ventilation

Ventilation

The next very important, big thing is ventilation. Ventilation refers to the movement of air in and out of the system as we both deliver breaths and allow exhalation. As discussed before, this is vitally important for the movement of carbon dioxide. Too much carbon dioxide hanging out in the lungs with no escape is bad news, so we can't just focus on getting oxygen in. And while we typically think of carbon dioxide in the context of acid-base analysis, recognize that there are a great many reasons to keep it well-controlled.[129] So how do we know if we are moving enough air for a given patient? There are two strategies here, and we will discuss them both in turn: calculated minute volume and end-tidal monitoring of carbon dioxide ($EtCO_2$).

If we math it out, our minute volume goal for the typical patient should be:[130]

$$MV \approx 100\text{ml/kg IBW/min}$$

This number varies a bit for patients with an increased need (i.e. **Acidosis**), but it's a good place to start as written and is an appropriate minimum for most patients. Having a goal minute ventilation in mind and then assessing actual minute volume (typically measured by the vent) is a great way to ensure that the patient's needs are met.

Concurrently, we also use $EtCO_2$ to monitor ventilation.[131] When the body uses up oxygen at the tissue level, it kicks back carbon dioxide into the bloodstream. That carbon dioxide then makes its way up to the lungs where it passes into the alveoli and then is exhaled out. It looks about opposite to our previous sketch showing how oxygen moves through the system:

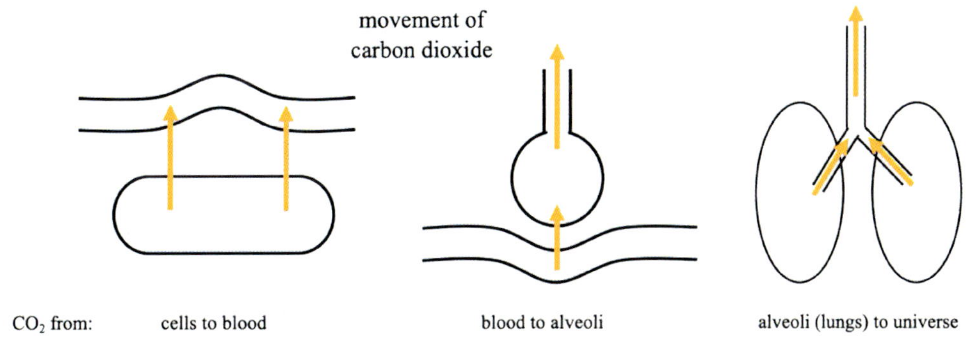

[129] Yartsev, 2019 – See this page for a very thorough overview of how carbon dioxide can affect the body in different ways
[130] We discussed where this minute volume goal number comes from previously (in the section titled **Minute Volume**); and see section on **Ideal Body Weight** to review the basis of this idea, that lung size best correlates with height
[131] Siobal, 2016 – We will cite this article again later (in **Acidosis** and in the **Appendix**), but it is an excellent resource for learning more about $EtCO_2$ monitoring and related concepts

CO_2 – carbon dioxide; **$EtCO_2$** – end-tidal carbon dioxide; **IBW** – ideal body weight; **kg** – kilogram; **min** – minute; **ml** – milliliter; **mmHg** – millimeters of mercury

The value we get on our quantitative $EtCO_2$ reading is a function of all of these factors. The standard approach to managing ventilation with $EtCO_2$ is to use a base range and adjust minute volume to get the value within that acceptable range. Normal range for $EtCO_2$ is 35-45mmHg; values above range require an increase in minute volume to blow off more carbon dioxide, values below that require us to read the next paragraph carefully.

A low $EtCO_2$ can be caused by a few different things, one of which is hyperventilation. This can be detrimental to a patient, as an alkalotic state (due to too much minute volume and a low $EtCO_2$) can throw off the patient's homeostasis. In this case, it'd make sense to decrease minute volume (by lowering either rate or tidal volume) to get the $EtCO_2$ (and therefore ventilation) back to normal. All that said, a low $EtCO_2$ could also be due to a breakdown somewhere else in the system (i.e. at any of those yellow lines in the previous drawing). For example, if perfusion is no good we may see a low $EtCO_2$ even though the issue is not necessarily a ventilation problem. In this case we could kill the patient by chasing their $EtCO_2$ or dropping minute volume to an unsustainable level.

We can navigate this whole situation by managing ventilation by looking at both minute volume and $EtCO_2$ instead of just $EtCO_2$. There are times when we will be a bit off with minute volume and others when our goal range for $EtCO_2$ varies, but this system of dual parameters to evaluate ventilation is a safety check to remind us of all the factors involved. To summarize: we measure ventilation using both a calculated minute volume goal and $EtCO_2$. This minute volume goal, which is considered a minimum in most cases, is around 100ml/kg IBW/min; normal $EtCO_2$ is 35-45mmHg.

And one final point before we move on: when faced with the choice as to whether we should manipulate **Respiratory Rate** or **Tidal Volume** to effect a change in **Minute Volume**, here's what we recommend: to increase minute volume, utilize tidal volume first; to decrease minute volume utilize rate first. Now we are going to outline an argument as to why that is and then follow up with some thoughts on why that rationale isn't quite as good as it is often presented to be. So hold with us through this explanation and then we'll discuss it afterwards. Know that the basis of the idea still holds true, it's mainly a matter of to what degree this difference actually exists in practice.

Let's say we have a patient breathing at a rate of 15 and a tidal volume of 450ml:

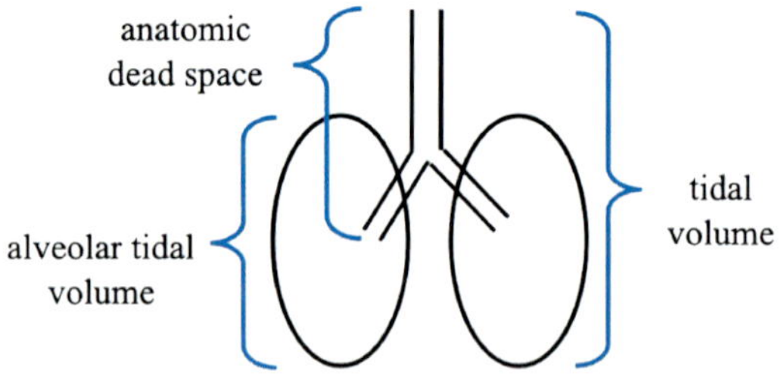

tidal volume 450ml		minute volume = 6750ml/min
- anatomic dead space 150ml	x 15/min	
alveolar tidal volume 300ml		alveolar minute volume = 4500ml/min

MV – minute volume; **O_2** – oxygen; **PEEP** – positive end-expiratory pressure; **VA** – alveolar minute ventilation

Now assume we want to increase alveolar minute volume by an arbitrary value of 300ml. We could do this by either of two ways: increasing rate to 16 or increasing the volume of each breath by 20ml. While either method is just fine mathematically, adding in an extra breath is a bit less efficient and puts more stress into the system. That stress comes in a few different forms, but we'll get to all of those later.[132] And here's how the math would look in either case:

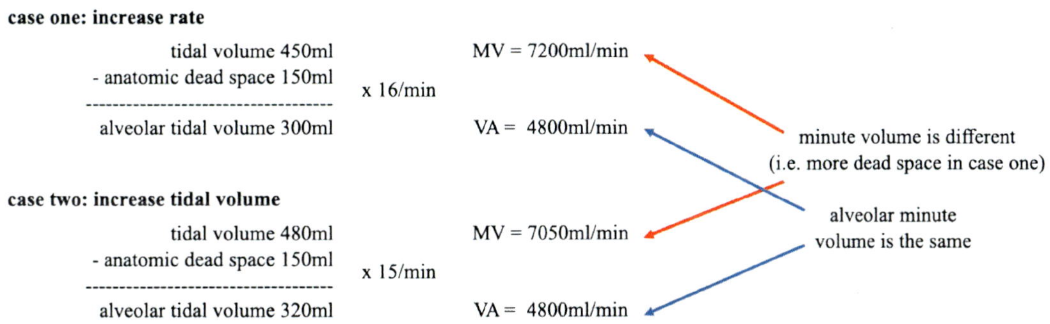

Now on the opposite end of things, if $EtCO_2$ is low (which indicates too much minute volume), then we back off on respiratory rate first. That gives us the same differences, but in the reverse: less alveolar minute volume (which is what we want) accompanied by less of the negative consequences. In reality, either strategy (titrating rate or tidal volume) is appropriate, it's just an extra thing to keep in mind if we want to be more resourceful in our vent changes.

While we've shown just now that it's more efficient to use tidal volume to increase ventilation and rate to decrease ventilation, know that both anatomic and alveolar dead space can sometimes increase with more tidal volume.[133] This means that the difference in both dead space and alveolar minute volume in the above calculations may not be as marked as we've demonstrated. The tough part about this is that we can't rightfully predict to what degree dead space will track with an increase in tidal volume, as there isn't a direct relationship between the two and it depends on a few other things: how the current tidal volume compares to overall lung capacity, how the breaths are being delivered, other vent settings (especially PEEP), concurrent disease processes, etc. So while we still recommend to consider the difference and use some discretion when making changes, know that this argument doesn't give the whole picture and that we can utilize rate or tidal volume to change minute volume in either direction.

And to summarize: ventilation is another one of the big things to address in mechanical ventilation. We start by using a weight-based goal for minute volume (by way of an age-based respiratory rate and weight-based tidal volume) and then titrate it as we go to an $EtCO_2$ goal. This minute volume goal is 100ml/kg IBW/min and a normal $EtCO_2$ is 35-45mmHg. More minute volume will drive $EtCO_2$ down, less minute volume will lead to an increase in $EtCO_2$. To increase minute volume, we go up on tidal volume and then rate; to decrease minute volume, we go down on rate and then tidal volume.

---

[132] More breaths means more of an impact on hemodynamic function (discussed in both **How is Positive-Pressure Ventilation Different?** and **Hypotension**) and an extra inflation/ deflation cycle which can put stress on the alveoli (discussed already in **Positive End-Expiratory Pressure** and again later on in **Driving Pressure**)

[133] Yartsev, 2019 – This page discusses the variation in dead space with changes in tidal volume; also refer back to the section on **Dead Space** if need be

AutoPEEP – intrinsic positive end-expiratory pressure; **EtCO2** – end-tidal carbon dioxide; **I:E** – inspiratory to expiratory

Comfort

The third very important parameter that we need to consider with vent management is patient comfort. On one hand, if our patient is not comfortable (i.e. fighting the vent or out of synch), then the therapeutic effects that we want will be more difficult to attain. This asynchrony can also lead to increased airway pressures (due to the development of **AutoPEEP**), which then leads to more problems downstream.[134] And one more thing: it's kind of rude to shove a plastic tube down someone's throat, take over their respiratory function in a way that goes opposite to normal physiology, and then load them up inside a small flying box with people crowded all around and lots of noise, vibration, weird lights, etc. So let's be nice people and keep our patient's feelings in mind.

When we manage comfort it is important to have a strategy for quantifying the idea so that we can gauge the efficacy of our interventions. Many agencies recommend scales or tools to use and here are some examples:

TABLE 3. RICHMOND AGITATION-SEDATION SCALE

Score	Term	Description
+4	Combative	Overtly combative or violent; immediate danger to staff
+3	Very agitated	Pulls on or removes tube(s) or catheter(s) or has aggressive behavior toward staff
+2	Agitated	Frequent nonpurposeful movement or patient-ventilator dyssynchrony
+1	Restless	Anxious or apprehensive but movements not aggressive or vigorous
0	Alert and calm	
−1	Drowsy	Not fully alert, but has sustained (more than 10 s) awakening, with eye contact in response to voice
−2	Light sedation	Briefly (less than 10 s) awakens with eye contact in response to voice
−3	Moderate sedation	Any movement (but no eye contact) in response to voice
−4	Deep sedation	No response to voice, but any movement in response to physical stimulation
−5	Unarousable	No response to voice or physical stimulation

Procedure

1.	Observe patient. Is patient alert and calm (score 0)?
	Does patient have behavior that is consistent with restlessness or agitation (score, +1 to +4 using the criteria listed under Description)?
2.	If patient is not alert, in a loud speaking voice state patient's name and direct patient to open eyes and look at speaker.
	Repeat once if necessary. Can prompt patient to continue looking at speaker.
	Patient has eye opening and eye contact, which is sustained for more than 10 s (score, −1)
	Patient has eye opening and eye contact, but this is not sustained for 10 s (score, −2)
	Patient has any movement in response to voice, excluding eye contact (score, −3)
3.	If patient does not respond to voice, physically stimulate patient by shaking shoulder and then rubbing sternum if there is no response to shaking shoulder.
	Patient has any movement to physical stimulation (score, −4)
	Patient has no response to voice or physical stimulation (score, −5)

Reprinted by permission from Reference 105.

[134] We first mentioned AutoPEEP in **Modes of Ventilation**, specifically when we talked about **Assist Control**

NVPS – nonverbal pain scale; **OK** – alright; **RASS** – Richmond agitation-sedation scale; **SIMV** – synchronized intermittent mandatory ventilation

TABLE 1. NONVERBAL PAIN SCALE

	Category		
	0	1	2
Face	No particular expression or smile	Occasional grimace, tearing, frowning, wrinkled forehead	Frequent grimace, tearing, frowning, wrinkled forehead
Activity (movement)	Lying quietly, normal position	Seeking attention through movement or slow, cautious movement	Restless, excessive activity and/or withdrawal reflexes
Guarding	Lying quietly, no positioning of hands over areas of body	Splinting areas of the body, tense	Rigid, stiff
Physiological I (vital signs)	Stable vital signs (no change in past 4 h)	Change over past 4 h in any of the following: SBP > 20 mm Hg, HR > 20 beats/min, RR > 10 breaths/min	Change over the past 4 h in any of the following: SBP > 30 mm Hg, HR > 25 beats/min, RR > 20 breaths/min
Physiological II	Warm, dry skin	Dilated pupils, perspiring, flushing	Diaphoretic, pallor

Definition of abbreviations: HR = heart rate; RR = respiratory rate; SBP = systolic blood pressure.

Reprinted by permission from Reference 15.

On the other hand, however, a completely sedated patient making no effort to breathe on his or her own suffers 100% of the negative consequences of positive-pressure ventilation.[135] Maintaining patient effort and supporting it appropriately with the machine decreases the degree of all those negative things we previously discussed, shortens clinical course,[136] and helps improve both **Ventilation** and **Oxygenation**.[137] Furthermore, having access to subjective feedback from the patient (effort to breath, movement, response to stimuli, etc.) allows us to better monitor whatever else is going on. Because of this, sedation to the point of no spontaneous effort to breathe (or even paralysis, for that matter) should be a last resort for nearly all ventilated patients; instead, we should attempt to maintain comfort to a controlled level by both analgesia and sedation (which, just to clarify, are two distinct concepts).[138]

---

[135] We discussed these consequences of mechanical ventilation in **How is Positive-Pressure Ventilation Different?**

[136] Ghamloush & Hill, 2013 – While this article focuses on SIMV and how we maybe ought to phase it out, it touches on the idea of synchrony in a general sense along the way

[137] Mauri & friends, 2017; Macintyre, 2014 – The first discusses how to navigate the benefits of spontaneous breathing in the vented patient with potential consequences; the second outlines how comfort can decrease oxygen consumption in the vented patient

[138] Patel & Kress, 2011 – This article outlines some thoughts on both analgesia and sedation in the vented patient; we've also taken the graphics for the NVPS and RASS scores from this article

AutoPEEP – intrinsic positive end-expiratory pressure; **$EtCO_2$** – end-tidal carbon dioxide; **I:E** – inspiratory to expiratory

Just to be clear, there are some patients who will need to be completely sedated and/ or paralyzed. In the transport setting, this often comes up in the context of safety concerns. A patient who has previously been difficult to restrain or who has already self-extubated once before may need to be paralyzed to ensure safe transport. There may also be the argument that breathing spontaneously or making the effort to do so increases oxygen consumption and could exacerbate certain conditions. So while we prefer not to paralyze anyone, it may very well be in his or her best interest for us to do so. Just remember that we will still need to consider discomfort (and pain in particular) and address it appropriately. In those cases, we can make a subjective impression about comfort by looking at physiologic changes as outlined on the bottom two lines of the NVPS score:

TABLE 1. NONVERBAL PAIN SCALE

	Category		
	0	1	2
Physiological I (vital signs)	Stable vital signs (no change in past 4 h)	Change over past 4 h in any of the following: SBP > 20 mm Hg, HR > 20 beats/min, RR > 10 breaths/min	Change over the past 4 h in any of the following: SBP > 30 mm Hg, HR > 25 beats/min, RR > 20 breaths/min
Physiological II	Warm, dry skin	Dilated pupils, perspiring, flushing	Diaphoretic, pallor

Definition of abbreviations: HR = heart rate; RR = respiratory rate; SBP = systolic blood pressure.

Now let's move on to differentiate between the ideas of synchrony and compliance. Synchrony is when the ventilator's efforts are in line with the patient's respiratory effort.[139] Asynchrony, therefore, would be when the patient wants a breath in a given instant, but the machine decides to give a breath some other time. Compliance, on the other hand, is used to describe how well the patient follows the lead of the ventilator.[140] A paralyzed patient is for sure compliant, but that doesn't mean it should be the goal we aim for. Rather we should strive for synchrony and let the patient take the lead on things, adjusting settings along the way to match mechanical support to patient cues.

The strategy to address comfort for the vented patient is to treat the extreme end of discomfort using drugs (both analgesia and sedation) and then do what we can to optimize synchrony on the vent itself once the patient is comfortable enough to respond to more fine-tuned settings. To begin this fine-tuning, we first want to make sure that patient effort to breathe is supported by the machine. We'll talk about **Triggers** later, but the general idea is that we don't want to ignore patient effort, and we also don't want to send breaths down the circuit accidentally. We may have to trial different thresholds and types of triggers until we find what best suits the patient and that's completely OK.

---

[139] Goligher, 2017 – This article (which we referenced before) is brief, but gets into the details on some of the more subtle concepts in this discussion of synchrony

[140] And this use of the term compliance to describe a patient following the ventilator's lead is different than the idea of lung compliance which we discuss later in **Compliance (and Resistance)**

NVPS – nonverbal pain scale; **OK** – alright; **RASS** – Richmond agitation-sedation scale; **SIMV** – synchronized intermittent mandatory ventilation

Another thing we can do is adjust **Inspiratory Time (and I:E Ratio)**. Occasionally a minor adjustment here can make a patient feel more comfortable. One thing to keep in mind is that a normal I:E ratio is 1:2 and that a larger ratio closer to 1:1 is common at exercise or exertion.[141] While the link from exercise to acute illness may not hold up in all cases, this helps explain how the lower ratios (1:3 and beyond) we commonly end up with on the vent (due to how settings get auto-calculated) may predispose our patient to discomfort. For example, if we start with an I:E ratio of 1:2 and then titrate rate down to accommodate a high $EtCO_2$ and don't simultaneously increase inspiratory time, we will have a smaller I:E ratio (again, 1:3 and beyond) that can be uncomfortable for our patient.

Switching mode or control may also help with discomfort. We mentioned this already, but different **Types of Breaths** are delivered differently in each mode or method of control, and sometimes one may work better for the patient. Discomfort is a completely valid reason to switch from volume control to pressure control (or vice versa) or to move from **Assist Control** to **Synchronized Intermittent Mandatory Ventilation** (again, or vice versa).[142] We will outline a few cases in which one style of ventilation may be preferred over another, but barring a specific reason not to do the swap this is one way we can attempt to address comfort by changing settings on the vent. And specifically to SIMV, if we have a patient triggering breaths we can go up on pressure support and see how (s)he responds. We mentioned already that it is the custom to have pressure support breaths be smaller than mandatory or assisted ones, but that doesn't have to be the rule.

Now let's summarize our approach to patient comfort, the third of the three big things to be addressed for all vented patients. Our goal in addressing comfort is to maximize synchrony and this includes both matching ventilator effort with patient need and maintaining the patient's spontaneous effort. To help gauge this all, a scoring system should be utilized. Extremes of discomfort get treated pharmacologically with both analgesia and sedation. After that, however, we can fine-tune ventilator settings to further maximize efficacy. Specific strategies include adjusting triggers, increasing inspiratory time to yield to a higher I:E ratio, trialing a different mode or method of control, and using higher values of pressure support if in SIMV mode.

---

[141] Johnston, 2017 – This page looks at this concept of I:E ratio with exertion in terms of a fraction of inspiratory time over expiratory time; while it is geared to pulmonary function tests and exercise physiology, it is still applicable to our discussion

[142] And refer back to **Modes of Ventilation** and **Control of Ventilation** to brush up on these ideas

Vent Parameters, Round Two

This next section discusses a few more vent parameters that we measure after the initial setup or taking over of a vented patient. They are considered separately from the values previously discussed because they are dependent on other things. We don't dial them into the machine, but rather we measure them to assess how things are coming along with the values we are able to control. To help clarify these ideas, let's refer back to an image we previously discussed. It shows pressure we put into the system over time as a breath is delivered in volume control ventilation:

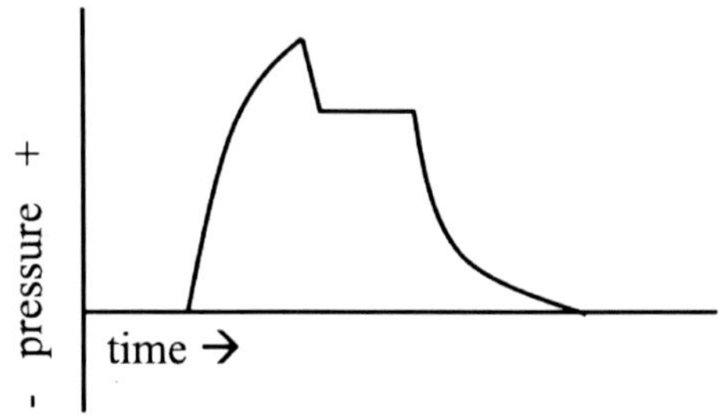

We previously used this graphic to demonstrate a couple of things, but it is now worth mentioning that this waveform and the two subsequent concepts (peak inspiratory pressure and plateau pressure) apply to volume control ventilation. Let's first get things clarified for volume control ventilation, and then we'll talk about how these concepts carry over into pressure control ventilation.

COPD – chronic obstructive pulmonary disease; **I:E** – inspiratory to expiratory; **OK** – alright; **PEEP** – positive end-expiratory pressure

Peak Inspiratory Pressure[143]

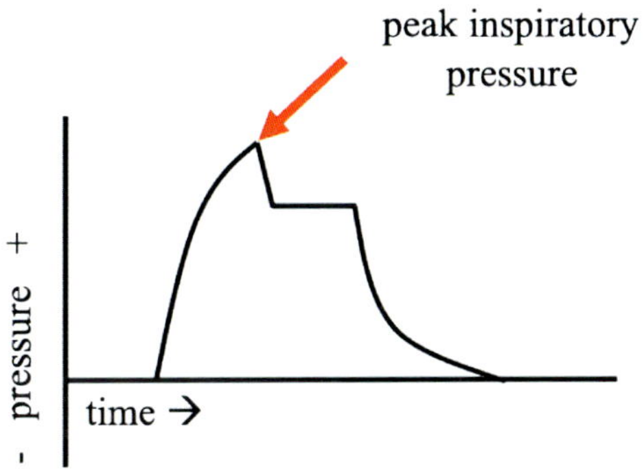

Peak inspiratory pressure (PIP) is the highest point on this waveform. It represents the maximum pressure as we deliver a breath into the system. It is also known as peak pressure (Ppeak). Peak inspiratory pressure is a function of both how we deliver a breath via the machine and how easily that breath can get from the machine down to the lungs. A normal peak inspiratory pressure is less than 35cmH_20. An isolated peak inspiratory pressure that is too high generally won't cause damage to the patient, rather it likely indicates something gone wrong in the system. This is particularly relevant when we have a normal peak pressure that then becomes elevated. In these cases it is important to seek out the cause and fix the underlying issue.

On the machine end, peak inspiratory pressure is the result of flow, which (recall from our section on **Types of Breaths**) essentially describes how fast we push air to achieve a breath. We sometimes can't manipulate flow directly on transport ventilators, so to decrease peak inspiratory pressure by pushing buttons on the machine we have to make things happen in a roundabout way. Which isn't ideal and the truth of it all is that most of the peak inspiratory pressure issues we face are due to pathophysiology or equipment issues, so let's just skip right on ahead to how we can decrease peak inspiratory pressure via other mechanisms outside of the vent itself.[144]

Causes of an elevated peak inspiratory pressure include things like secretions in the endotracheal tube, bronchospasm, patient discomfort, mainstem intubation, pneumothorax, pulmonary edema, etc. Any time we see a high peak inspiratory pressure we ought to try and identify a cause.[145] Once that cause is identified, then we can decide whether or not an action is needed. For example, a high peak pressure due to secretions should get suction and a high peak pressure due to a pneumothorax should lead to decompression; on the other hand, a high peak pressure due to a small endotracheal tube may be acceptable. The peak inspiratory pressure in this last case represents an impediment to airflow due to the tube and not the patient's anatomy, so we may decide to leave it alone (especially is there is good reason for that small endotracheal tube, such as airway swelling).

---

[143] Nickson, 2019a – Short article that provides another good review of both peak inspiratory pressure (this section) and plateau pressure (next section); cited normal values are supported by his content

[144] But for the curious folks out there: in volume control flow is determined from tidal volume and inspiratory time; in pressure control (and with pressure support breaths) it is a function of pressure and rise time

[145] And one part of how to identify the cause of a high peak inspiratory is by assessing **Plateau Pressure** (next section); we have this all drawn out in a flowchart later, but first we need discuss all the terms and concepts first (see **Watching Pressures**)

ΔP –driving pressure; **AutoPEEP** – intrinsic positive end-expiratory pressure; **cmH_2O** – centimeters of water

Another consideration here is patient comfort and the idea of laminar flow. Without getting too far into this, recognize that air can move freely and efficiently through a uniform pipe or tube, but with movement or disruption to that tube, airflow will be more chaotic and result in higher pressures. Keeping our patient comfortable and in synch with the vent leads to more uniform (i.e. efficient) air movement and lower peak pressure. Takeaway here: make sure our vented patient is comfortable. And if we notice an increase in peak inspiratory pressure, **Comfort** ought to be one of the things to consider.

To measure peak inspiratory pressure we simply need to look at the vent display. Most machines will either give us the value or show a barometer that fluctuates with each breath. Peak inspiratory pressure is always the highest value that comes up during a breath. Another way to keep an eye on peak pressure is by setting an alarm so that machine yells at us when a certain pressure is reached. That said, there is one critical thing to know about this: yes it will tell us that the pressure has gotten too high, but it will likely (depending on model) also cycle off the breath it is giving in response to that high-pressure alarm. This can potentially kill our patient and we will get into that a bit more later on.[146]

So in summary, peak inspiratory pressure represents the maximum pressure as a breath is delivered by the machine. A normal value is less than $35cmH_20$ and we measure it by looking at the feedback on the vent interface. Potential causes include too much air, too much flow, small or kinked endotracheal tube, patient discomfort, secretions, pneumothorax, mainstem tube placement, and bronchospasm. While there are subtle ways to address a high peak pressure that develops after placing a patient on the vent, interventions should focus instead on airway issues and comfort.

[146] This discussion of how breaths can get terminated early with the triggering of a high-pressure alarm is in the section on **Alarms**

COPD – chronic obstructive pulmonary disease; **I:E** – inspiratory to expiratory; **OK** – alright; **PEEP** – positive end-expiratory pressure

Plateau Pressure

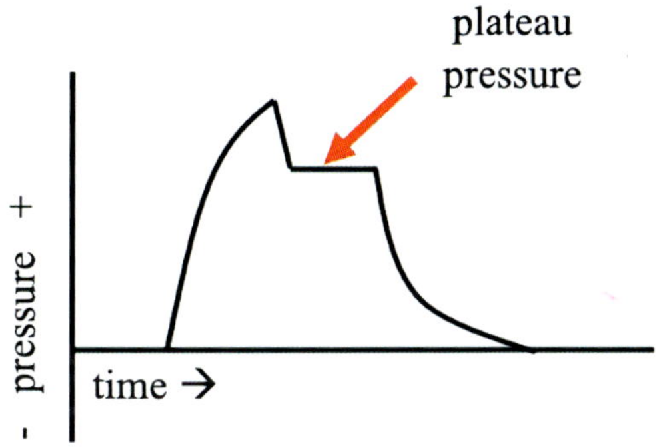

Plateau pressure (Pplat) is the pressure in the system once the lungs are filled with air and before the breath cycles off. It represents the average pressure at the alveoli as they are at maximum inflation during inhalation. A normal plateau pressure is less than 30cm$H_2 0$. Values higher than that can lead to direct damage to the alveoli, which can subsequently cause issues with pulmonary respiration.[147] There is no minimum or lower limit for plateau pressure, but recognize that lungs that aren't being filled all the way (i.e. a low plateau pressure) may not be maximizing the surface area of alveoli and therefore **Oxygenation** may not be at its best. And we will discuss this concept later on.[148]

The primary cause of a high plateau pressure at the start of ventilation is too much **Tidal Volume**. That said, it can also be present or develop over time due to patient discomfort, mainstem migration of the endotracheal tube, atelectasis, and pulmonary edema. If we get a high plateau pressure, consider these other causes (and address them appropriately) before dialing down tidal volume, as we don't want to give up ventilation unnecessarily.[149] We do, however, want to avoid a sustained high plateau pressure over many breaths, as that can lead to damage to the alveoli.

Measuring plateau pressure is a little less direct than measuring peak inspiratory pressure and involves what we call a maneuver. There are two maneuvers that we will discuss and this is the first of them. While we could theoretically watch the barometer on the machine and wait for that point during inspiration where pressure stays constant for a spell, that amount of time is quite short and this is logistically difficult to accomplish. The workaround is to prolong inspiration via an inspiratory hold and allow the machine to measure that pressure accurately. It would look something like this:

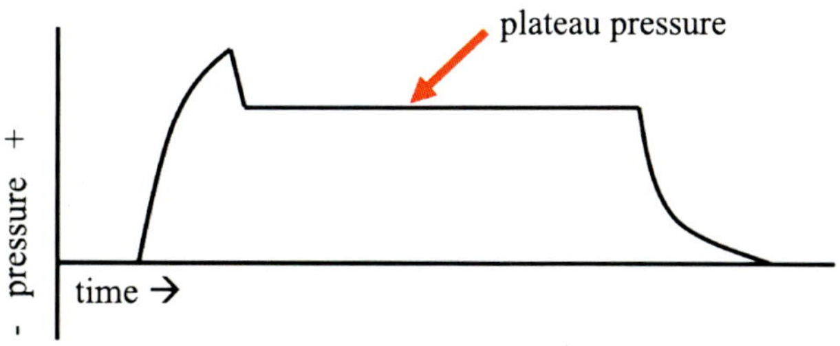

[147] We defined this concept of pulmonary respiration back in **Terms to Describe Breathing**

[148] In **Titrating Up on Tidal Volume?** we will review thoughts on how to address a low plateau pressure

[149] We revisit this idea of managing abnormal airway pressures in an algorithmic fashion in the section called **Watching Pressures**

ΔP –driving pressure; **AutoPEEP** – intrinsic positive end-expiratory pressure; **cmH_2O** – centimeters of water

We perform the inspiratory hold maneuver (in whatever way is appropriate for our particular machine) and the plateau pressure either pops up on the screen for us or we have enough time to read the value from the barometer. Easy enough, but when and how often do we do this thing? There isn't a universally accepted frequency for measuring this (or any of the other pressures discussed in this section), but it seems to make sense that we just add them on to our reassessment of vital signs (so every 5-15 minutes, depending on the program and patient acuity). While that may be overkill, it's better to measure too much than to miss things due to not checking often enough. At a minimum, plateau pressure should be measured after any increase in tidal volume to make sure that we don't cause alveolar damage (and this includes after first putting the patient on the vent).

Another thing about plateau pressure is that the value we get is an average of alveolar pressures across the lung - some regions will experience higher pressures and others will experience lower pressures. The lung is not uniform throughout, but we can't measure alveolar pressures in specific lung regions or see to what degree this value would vary across the different parts. The safe limit of less than $30cmH_2O$ is a good guideline by which to limit our vent settings, but recognize that this doesn't mean that a pressure higher than that to one alveolus or a region of the lung will always cause harm. Likewise, a plateau pressure below $30cmH_2O$ is not a guarantee that damage will not be caused.

One more subtlety here is that an elevated plateau pressure doesn't always reflect stress on the alveoli, there may be something external to the alveoli that prevents them from opening:

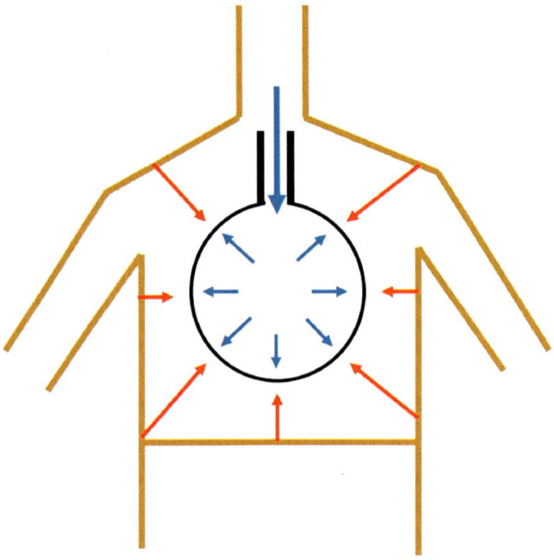

In these cases the elevated plateau pressure is not due to distention at the alveoli, rather it is due to something else. Examples would be a tension pneumothorax, burn to the chest wall, or even physical compression as with an entrapped patient. So while we generalize plateau pressure as a reflection of alveolar pressure, know that this isn't always the case.

In summary, plateau pressure is typically the pressure seen by the alveoli when we deliver a breath in volume control ventilation. A normal value is less than $30cmH_20$ and we measure it by performing an inspiratory hold maneuver. While there is no bottom limit to plateau pressure, it is important to recognize that we want to fill the lung and alveoli up with each breath delivered, so be wary of a super low plateau pressure and consider inadequate tidal volume (and subsequently minute volume). High plateau pressure can be caused by too much tidal volume, pneumothorax, restriction to chest wall expansion, mainstem intubation, and a few other things that we'll spell out later on.

COPD – chronic obstructive pulmonary disease; **I:E** – inspiratory to expiratory; **OK** – alright; **PEEP** – positive end-expiratory pressure

Airway Pressures in Pressure Control?

Up to this point we've discussed **Peak Inspiratory Pressure** and **Plateau Pressure** in the context of **Volume Control** ventilation, but things are a bit different in **Pressure Control**. Let's start with what a pressure control breath looks like mapped out as pressure over time:[150]

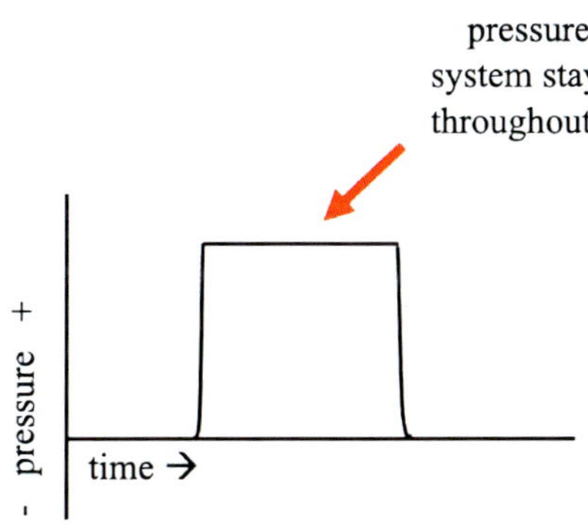

First thing to mention here is that the top of that waveform (i.e. the flat part) represents the value we have set for pressure control and that we often refer to that value as peak inspiratory pressure. For example, we could either say that the patient is in pressure control with a pressure control of X or that the patient is in pressure control with a peak pressure of X. Either way is just fine. The only caveat here is to consider if that pressure control value is additive to or inclusive of PEEP (as we discussed in **Types of Breaths**). Peak inspiratory pressure is always an absolute value that represents a pressure measured against the atmosphere.

Since the machine in pressure control limits pressure into the system, the actual highest pressure will only be above that flat line at the top of the square waveform (marked by the red arrow in the graphic) if something causes a disturbance in what the machine is doing, such as a hiccup, patient movement, speedbump, etc. The machine won't intentionally put more pressure than what we have set, but a peak pressure higher than the set pressure control can occur. So while we may still set a high-pressure alarm and monitor peak inspiratory pressure in pressure control ventilation, our concern is more for being aware of disturbances to the system rather than being aware of changes to airflow, as was the case in volume control ventilation.[151]

[150] To review these types of waveforms and how this pressure control waveform differs from a volume control one, refer back to **Types of Breaths**

[151] In pressure control ventilation, we become aware of those obstruction issues by monitoring exhaled tidal volume (and maybe flow, if available on our particular machine)

ΔP –driving pressure; **AutoPEEP** – intrinsic positive end-expiratory pressure; **cmH_2O** – centimeters of water

Next thing: the goal is that the average alveolar pressure eventually does equal that pressure represented by the top of the square waveform (towards the end of expiration), therefore we assume it to be true that pressure control equals plateau pressure.[152] And because of this assumption that mostly holds true, it's OK that some machines don't let us do inspiratory holds in pressure control ventilation, as the data gleaned from the test just wouldn't provide any additional information. And also because the primary reason we want the plateau pressure (in volume control) is to rule out high alveolar pressures (to ensure the wellbeing of the alveoli); in pressure control if plateau pressure doesn't match pressure control it's because true plateau pressure is less than the pressure control (which is a bummer, but not a safety concern for the alveoli).

Now the way it works is that it takes time for the alveolar pressure to rise up to match the pressure going into the system. Even though we start with a high pressure at the machine end of the system, it may take some time for that pressure to equalize down to the alveoli. If our **Inspiratory Time** isn't long enough to allow that to happen, the alveolar pressure may not ever get up to the level we have set for pressure control. We work around that in volume control by performing an inspiratory hold and waiting for as long as we need to in order to see that pressure even out. We don't always do that in pressure control because, as we said just a moment ago, the **Plateau Pressure** won't be above our pressure control value and it isn't so much of a concern.

But if we wanted to know a little more about what's going on in the alveoli and we can't do an inspiratory hold on our machine in pressure control, we can get a partial picture of things by looking at flow. Pressure control breaths start with a higher flow that then drops down towards zero throughout the breath. While it may be hard to see with quantitative values on our machine (unless we can view waveforms), if flow doesn't get down to zero before the breath cycles off, then we can consider that the pressure in the alveoli may not have made it up to the level we put in on the front end:

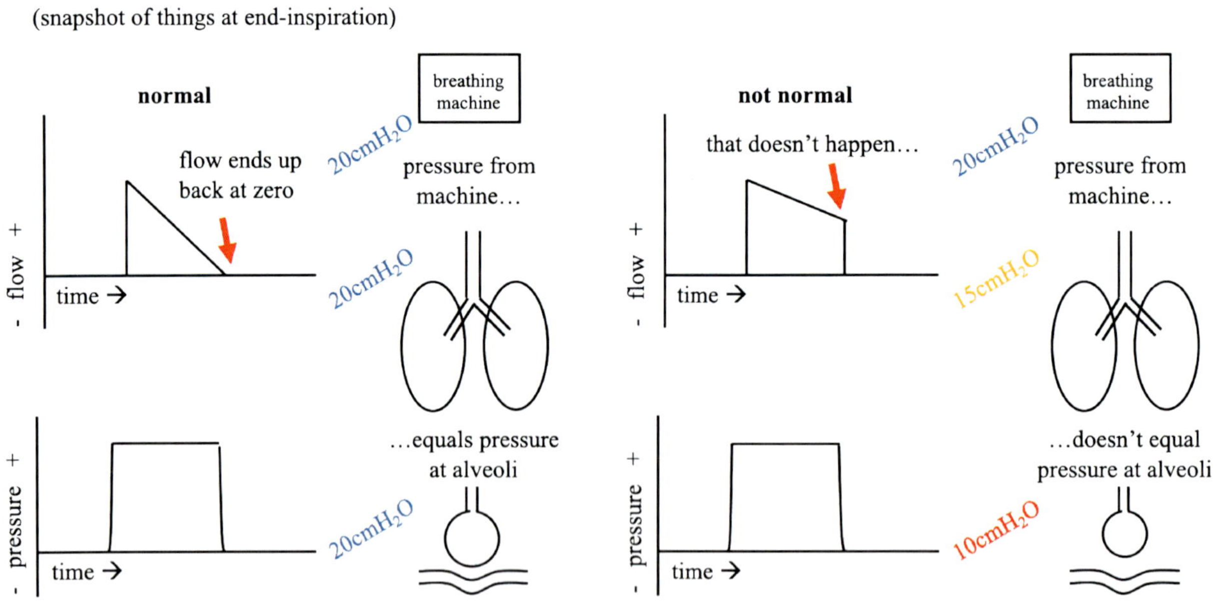

---

[152] Hess, 2014 – Another way to say this is that if flow gets to zero during the inspiratory phase, then peak inspiratory pressure equals plateau pressure

COPD – chronic obstructive pulmonary disease; **I:E** – inspiratory to expiratory; **OK** – alright; **PEEP** – positive end-expiratory pressure

All that said, this isn't a great method unless we have waveforms to look at. And even then it's a binary thing. It says whether or not alveolar pressure got up to the value of pressure control, but it doesn't tell us what the alveolar pressure actually was. There are other ways to measure or approximate plateau pressure, although they are unlikely to be available to us in the transport setting.[153]

So what utility is there in knowing plateau pressure in pressure control anyways? We said already that the usefulness of this information in volume control is to prevent damage to the alveoli, but that isn't as much of an issue in pressure control. Potential uses of knowing a plateau pressure in pressure control would be making sure our inspiratory time is appropriate (i.e. that the inspiratory time is long enough to allow pressure going in to match pressure at the alveoli) and calculating things like compliance and driving pressure (both discussed later).[154] These are all cool things to work with, but it takes both time and effort and, therefore, may not be the best use of one's cognitive capacity when managing a sick patient in the transport setting. We will discuss this stuff, but know that plateau pressure is primarily a tool for ensuring alveolar safety in volume control ventilation.

AutoPEEP

AutoPEEP is the idea of **Positive End-Expiratory Pressure** being cumulatively added into the system inadvertently. It is also known as intrinsic PEEP. Remember how we said that we assume atmospheric pressure to be $0cmH_20$ as the starting point for our vent discussions and that PEEP is the addition of pressure on top of that (i.e. "adding 5cm of PEEP" to reset that baseline to $5cmH_20$)? Well, AutoPEEP is when that baseline starts to creep up from whatever we have set as PEEP to higher values because the patient isn't able to exhale all the way back to baseline before the next breath comes around. This idea is commonly referred to as breath stacking and can be represented like this:

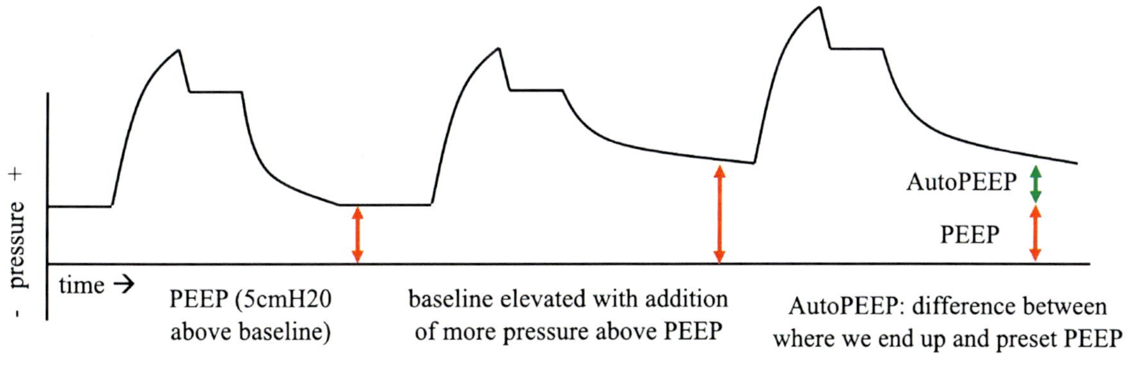

[153] Mojoli & friends, 2015 –This short paper assesses the efficacy of these alternative methods of measuring plateau pressure
[154] In the sections **Compliance (and Resistance)** and **Driving Pressure**

ΔP –driving pressure; **AutoPEEP** – intrinsic positive end-expiratory pressure; **cmH₂O** – centimeters of water

Normal AutoPEEP is zero, which means we shouldn't have any AutoPEEP in the system at all. That said, we may be OK with a few cmH_2O worth of AutoPEEP before we take action. Presence of AutoPEEP in **Volume Control** can lead to an increase in other airway pressures, most importantly of which is **Plateau Pressure**:

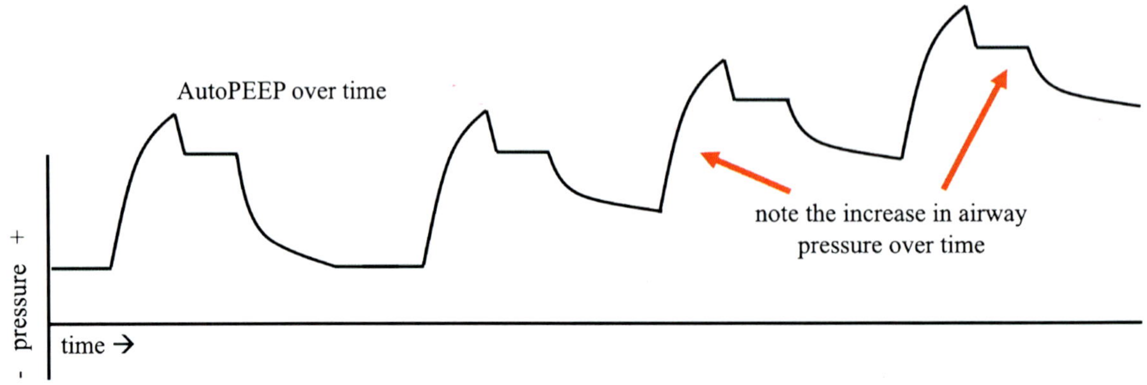

Another thing to realize is that if we have a normally-set high-pressure limit in place, then **Minute Volume** will suffer as breaths get terminated early:[155]

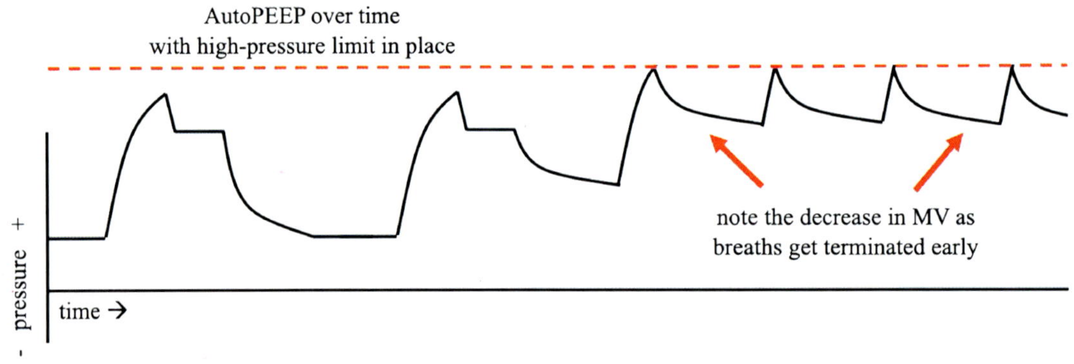

[155] We talk about this high-pressure alarm and the fact that it can compromise minute volume later on in **Alarms**

COPD – chronic obstructive pulmonary disease; **I:E** – inspiratory to expiratory; **OK** – alright; **PEEP** – positive end-expiratory pressure

AutoPEEP in **Pressure Control** will also result in decreased minute volume (due to less exhaled tidal volume per breath), but by a slightly different mechanism. Breaths don't get cut short as they do in volume control, rather the flow to get to that set pressure is less. And since volume delivered is the product of flow and time, we get less volume:[156]

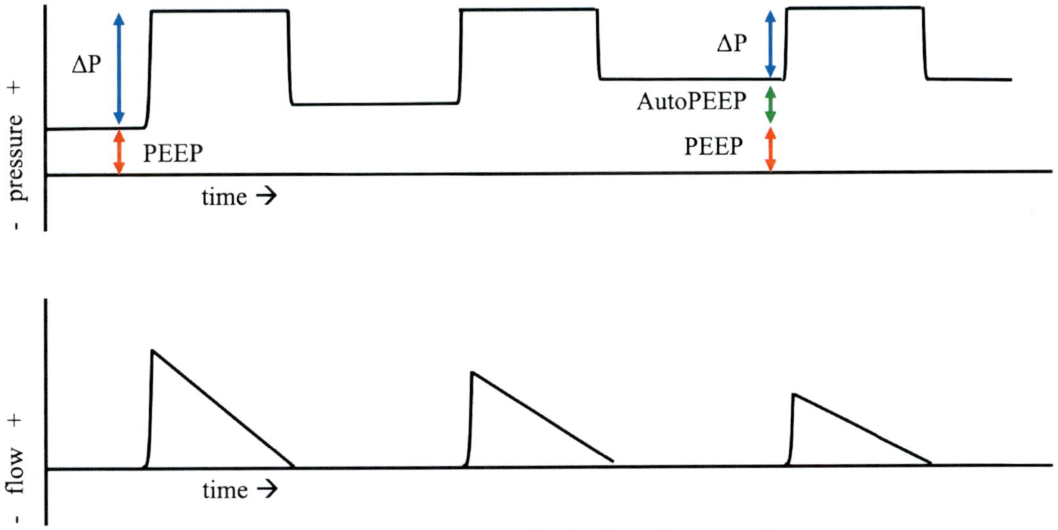

tidal volume = area under the flow time waveform
less ΔP = less flow required = less tidal volume

To measure AutoPEEP or to check its presence, we have to perform another maneuver called an expiratory hold.[157] Doing an expiratory hold allows us to accurately see what the pressure is when we expect the breath to have returned to baseline. Normally the machine will calculate an AutoPEEP for us by subtracting PEEP from whatever pressure it measures during the hold.

If we do have AutoPEEP, this means that something is getting in the way of the patient exhaling all the way back to baseline before a subsequent breath is delivered. This could be due to patient discomfort or need for more minute volume, but it can also be due to obstructive processes that get in the way of effective exhalation (i.e. asthma and COPD) or even inadvertent triggering of breaths. The fix on the vent interface would be to shorten our inspiratory time or decrease rate to lengthen the expiratory time (decrease the I:E ratio) and allow more exhalation; otherwise we could consider more sedation/ pain control and make sure we aren't accidentally triggering.[158] There is also the idea of utilizing applied PEEP to mitigate AutoPEEP and we'll touch on this idea later when we talk about an **Obstruction** strategy.[159]

---

[156] We used the symbol ΔP to represent the difference between pressure control and (Auto)PEEP, this is also the notation for a concept known as **Driving Pressure** which we will get to in just a bit

[157] There are other ways to check for AutoPEEP, but they aren't typically available in transport unless we have access to waveforms

[158] See sections on **Comfort**, **Triggers**, **Inspiratory Time (and I:E Ratio)**, **Types of Breaths**, and **Obstruction** for more on these things

[159] Stather & Stewart, 2005 – And for a preview of this idea (utilizing PEEP to mitigate AutoPEEP), refer to this article

ΔP –driving pressure; **AutoPEEP** – intrinsic positive end-expiratory pressure; **cmH₂O** – centimeters of water

One other thing we can do to eliminate AutoPEEP and reestablish our baseline at actual PEEP is to disconnect the patient from the vent circuit to allow a full and complete exhalation.[160] This is one of those rare cases in which it is OK to disconnect the vent circuit from the patient during transport for therapeutic reasons. Simply allow the patient to exhale and then reattach the circuit (and most likely canceling out a bunch of **Alarms** in the meantime). Just to make sure we understand how this works, let's draw it out as a waveform over time and label things along the way:

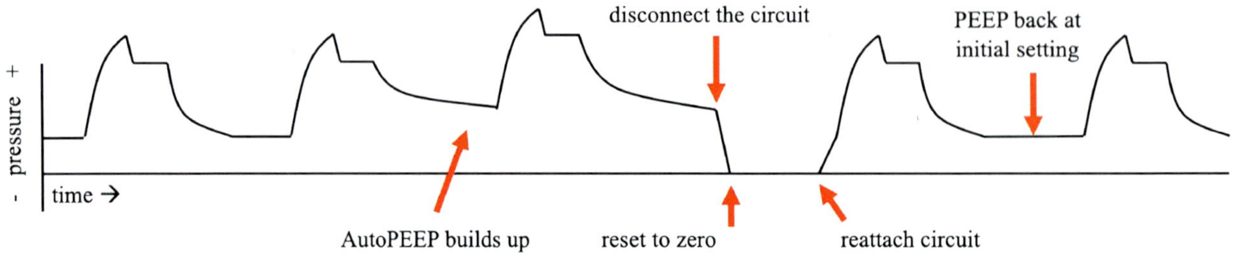

To summarize, AutoPEEP is a movement of the pressure baseline above whatever we have dialed in for PEEP. While a small amount of AutoPEEP may be tolerable, its presence is always an abnormal finding. Issues with this are increased pressures (volume control) or decreased volumes (both volume control and pressure control). Causes would be the inability to exhale fully, discomfort, and inadvertent triggering. Fixes include lengthening the expiratory time (decreasing I:E ratio), treating discomfort, avoiding accidental triggers, and utilizing applied PEEP. In addition, we can reset AutoPEEP back to zero by temporarily disconnecting the vent circuit.

[160] Do note that there are some patients in which disconnecting the circuit probably isn't the best option, this is mainly a concern with **Lung Injury** when we are particularly concerned with recruitment of alveoli

COPD – chronic obstructive pulmonary disease; **I:E** – inspiratory to expiratory; **OK** – alright; **PEEP** – positive end-expiratory pressure

Mean Airway Pressure

Last pressure to talk about is mean airway pressure. It's typically represented as P_{aw} (stands for airway pressure), sometimes as Pmean (mean pressure), and less often as MAP (mean airway pressure).[161] Mean airway pressure is the average pressure in the system throughout the respiratory cycle. There are formulas to estimate mean airway pressure, but it's probably easiest to just read off of our machine (assuming it's there).[162] We don't often use this pressure to guide treatment, but if we notice changes in mean airway pressure we can then look in to details as to what changed in the system. For example, a high mean airway pressure can result from all sorts of things, each of which is a totally different issue: an increase in either **Peak Inspiratory Pressure** or **Plateau Pressure**, the presence of **AutoPEEP**, and increased **Respiratory Rate**. And same thing on the opposite end, lots of things can cause mean airway pressure to drop and we then must work to identify a specific cause.

One other thing about mean airway pressure is that it is strongly correlated with **Oxygenation**, particularly due to the variables of **Positive End-Expiratory Pressure** and **Inspiratory Time**.[163] More of either of these things leads to a higher mean airway pressure, so it can help to think of oxygenation in terms of this pressure and **Fraction of Inspired Oxygen**. Just recognize that too much of this good thing can turn bad (i.e. too much pressure can lead to poor outcomes, as previously discussed). And while we commonly separate oxygenation into multiple concepts (as we did previously), it may be worth keeping this in mind as we look for trends in patient presentation:

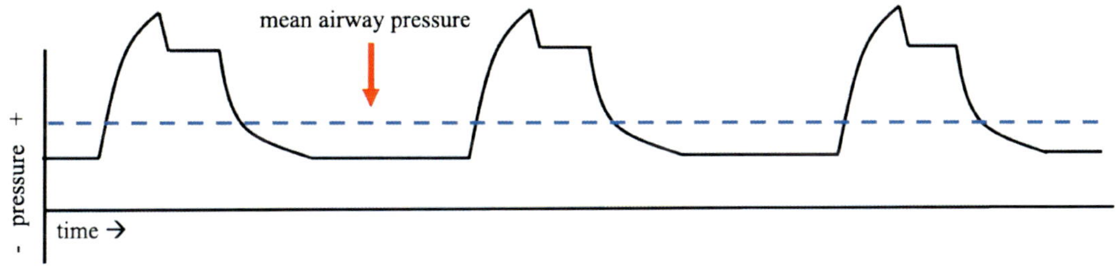

[161] And P_{aw} sometimes is used for airway pressure in general (i.e. the y-axis in the graphic on this page is airway pressure and that value changes throughout the breath), but we'll stick with it as a symbol for mean airway pressure in this manual

[162] We use one of these formulas to estimate mean airway pressure in the **Appendix** in order to demonstrate something about a **Hypotension** strategy we will outline later

[163] Lodeserto, 2018 – This page provides an alternative explanation for this relationship between mean airway pressure and oxygenation

ARDS – acute respiratory distress syndrome; **cmH_2O** – centimeters of water; **$EtCO_2$** – end-tidal carbon dioxide; **FiO_2** – fraction of inspired oxygen; **IBW** – ideal body weight; **I-time** – inspiratory time; **kg** – kilogram; **L** – liter; **ml** – milliliter; **min** – minute; **MV** – minute volume

A General Vent Strategy

In this section we are going to summarize general parameters in each type of ventilation (i.e. each combination of mode and control) in order to demonstrate what settings and goals are shared among all methods and which are specific to certain types of ventilation. This general strategy is similar to what is often described as a lung-protective strategy that first came on the scene in regard to management of patients with ARDS. We've opted to present the two as distinct strategies and we'll come back to this idea when we get there.[164] We will also hash out a few of the differences in determining general settings for adults versus pediatrics. Let's start with a discussion of things that apply to most vented patients, regardless of mode or control:[165]

$$TV = 6 - 8\text{ml/kg IBW}$$
$$MV \approx 100\text{ml/kg IBW /min}$$

if we choose a tidal volume of 6ml/kg and our goal minute volume is 100ml/kg/min, then our calculated respiratory rate is 17:

$$MV = RR \times TV$$
$$100\text{ml/kg/min} = RR \times 6\text{ml/kg}$$
$$100\cancel{\text{ml/kg}}\text{/min} \div 6\cancel{\text{ml/kg}} = RR$$
$$17 \approx RR$$

Likewise, if we go with 8ml/kg our initial rate (to match that minute volume goal) comes to 13 per minute. Although it's not uncommon to see recommendations for an initial rate of 10 to 12 with adults, calculating a rate based on a minute volume goal is our preferred strategy. There are often good reasons to use a lower rate, but we'll get to those later.[166]

Moving forward, if we have a range of tidal volume to choose from, sometimes it just makes life easier to pick a nice, even number. For example, with an 80kg patient we end up with a tidal volume goal range of 480-640ml and a minute volume goal of 8L; it's a totally legit move to choose 500 or 600 or any value in that range. Just recognize that if we pick a higher value for tidal volume, we want a lower value for respiratory rate just to keep our minute volume approximately the same. This does not have to be exact, as we will adjust these settings as we go and work towards our goals moving forward. So we may choose a tidal volume of 500 and a rate of 16 (for a calculated minute volume of 8L). Or a tidal volume of 600 and a rate of 14 (for a calculated minute volume of 8.4L). Either is cool for now and we'll dial in our settings once we see how the patient responds to it all.

---

[164] We discuss the management of ARDS in the section on **Lung Injury**

[165] Note that some patients do require different goals and we will discuss those shortly in **Specific Vent Strategies**; also, refer back to sections on **Tidal Volume**, **Ideal Body Weight**, **Respiratory Rate**, and **Minute Volume** for a discussion of these suggestions

[166] Specific examples of when we'd want to decrease rate below a normal range would be **Hypotension** and **Obstruction**

OK – alright; **PALS** – pediatric advances life support; **PEEP** – positive end-expiratory pressure; **PRVC** – pressure-regulated volume control; **RR** – respiratory rate; **s** – second; **SIMV** – synchronized intermittent mandatory ventilation; **TV** – tidal volume

As for kids, the approach is to choose a rate in line with a reference card and disregard the above suggestion of 13-17/min. While this will result in an overestimation of minute volume, we can titrate values to address that later on.[167] For example, let's assume a 4-year-old child of 18kg. Based on this chart (again, from PALS) we want a rate in the 20-28/min range:[168]

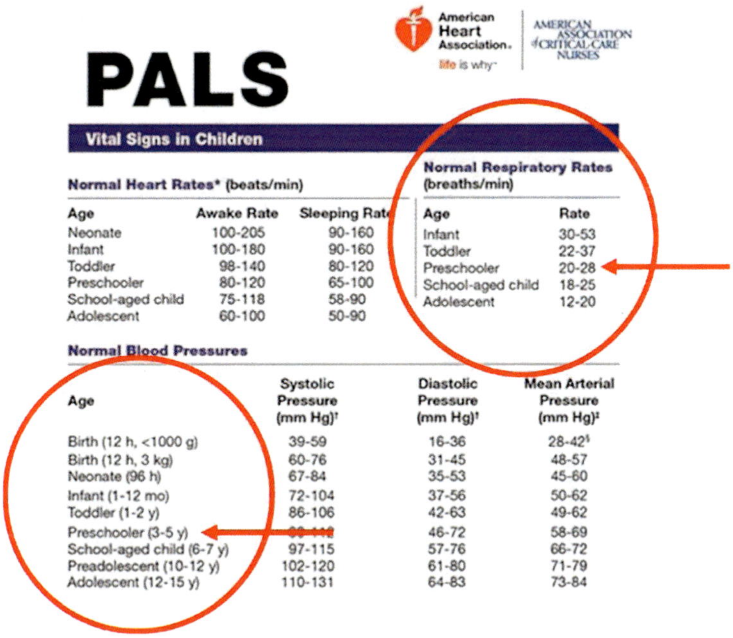

PALS

American Heart Association. life is why

AMERICAN ASSOCIATION of CRITICAL-CARE NURSES

Vital Signs in Children

Normal Heart Rates* (beats/min)

Age	Awake Rate	Sleeping Rate
Neonate	100-205	90-160
Infant	100-180	90-160
Toddler	98-140	80-120
Preschooler	80-120	65-100
School-aged child	75-118	58-90
Adolescent	60-100	50-90

Normal Respiratory Rates (breaths/min)

Age	Rate
Infant	30-53
Toddler	22-37
Preschooler	20-28
School-aged child	18-25
Adolescent	12-20

Normal Blood Pressures

Age	Systolic Pressure (mm Hg)†	Diastolic Pressure (mm Hg)†	Mean Arterial Pressure (mm Hg)‡
Birth (12 h, <1000 g)	39-59	16-36	28-42§
Birth (12 h, 3 kg)	60-76	31-45	48-57
Neonate (96 h)	67-84	35-53	45-60
Infant (1-12 mo)	72-104	37-56	50-62
Toddler (1-2 y)	86-106	42-63	49-62
Preschooler (3-5 y)	[illegible]	46-72	58-69
School-aged child (6-7 y)	97-115	57-76	66-72
Preadolescent (10-12 y)	102-120	61-80	71-79
Adolescent (12-15 y)	110-131	64-83	73-84

We can also use this chart based on the PALS data:[169]

age description	age (years)	rate	I-time (s)
infant	.083 (1 month) – 1	30 – 53	0.3 – 0.7
toddler	1 – 2	22 – 37	0.4 – 0.9
preschooler	3 – 5	22 – 28	0.5 – 0.9
school-aged child	6 – 7	18 – 25	0.6 – 1.1
big kids	8 – 9	17 – 25	0.6 – 1.2
preadolescent	10 – 12	14 – 23	0.7 – 1.4
adolescent	12 – 15	12 – 20	0.8 – 1.7
adult	16 and up	12 – 20	0.8 – 1.7

[167] This overestimation of minute volume is because we use a higher respiratory rate for pediatrics, but still utilize a weight-based tidal volume (or tidal volume goal in pressure control)

[168] American Heart Association, 2016 (image)

[169] As we mentioned before, see **Appendix** for an explanation of how we made this chart for normal respiratory rates and inspiratory times by age

ARDS – acute respiratory distress syndrome; **cmH_2O** – centimeters of water; **$EtCO_2$** – end-tidal carbon dioxide; **FiO_2** – fraction of inspired oxygen; **IBW** – ideal body weight; **I-time** – inspiratory time; **kg** – kilogram; **L** – liter; **ml** – milliliter; **min** – minute; **MV** – minute volume

And let's take these values and do a few calculations as so:

$$TV = 6 - 8ml/kg\ IBW$$
$$TV = 6 - 8ml/kg \times 18kg$$
$$TV = 108 - 144ml$$

$$MV\ goal = 100ml/kg\ IBW/min$$
$$MV\ goal = 1800ml/min$$
$$MV\ goal = 1.8L/min$$

$$MV\ calculated = RR \times TV$$
$$MV\ calculated = (20 - 28)/min \times (108 - 144)ml$$
$$MV\ calculated = 2160 - 4032ml/min$$
$$MV\ calculated \approx 2 - 4L/min$$

The result here is a minute volume goal that differs pretty significantly from the calculated minute volume, but what to do with this information? We will eventually want a minute volume (preferably measured as exhaled minute volume) that matches or exceeds our quantitative goal of 100ml/kg/min and also gives us an $EtCO_2$ in the normal 35-45 range, but let's start with 6-8ml/kg anyways and work towards that goal in the first little while after starting ventilation. This overestimation is particularly important, and maybe even lifesaving, if we decide to ventilate a child in volume control. There is always some dead space that we introduce into the system and this overestimation will help to mitigate that. Along those same lines, it may also be worth using a tidal volume on the higher end of the range (again, this is only for kids in volume control ventilation) to further mitigate this effect.[170]

[170] For more on this idea of why we might want to use a tidal volume towards the higher end of normal for pediatrics, refer to the **Appendix**

OK – alright; **PALS** – pediatric advances life support; **PEEP** – positive end-expiratory pressure; **PRVC** – pressure-regulated volume control; **RR** – respiratory rate; **s** – second; **SIMV** – synchronized intermittent mandatory ventilation; **TV** – tidal volume

So we have tidal volume, minute volume, and respiratory rate all sorted, both for adults and kids. Next we need to consider the other parameters that are constant between modes and control methods. Let's put it into a chart just to make it easier to visualize. And this chart is basically a summary of the section **Vent Parameters, Round One**:

parameter	value	pro tips
TV	6-8ml/kg	pick an easy number to work with that falls in that range
MV	100ml/kg/min	just take IBW in kg and move the decimal over (75kg IBW = 7.5L MV goal)
RR	adult: 13-17/min kids: use a chart	carry a reference card or have an app on a device to quickly reference the pediatric values[171]
FiO_2	1.0, then titrate down	we can titrate down in big jumps also, no need to go in small increments unless we have good reason to do so[172]
PEEP	5-6cmH_2O	for most vents this will be whatever the machine defaults to
I-time	adult: 0.8-1.7s kids: use a chart	normal for the adult is 1.0s

[171] Pedi STAT – Great resource for quickly referencing pediatric doses and equipment sizes

[172] Weingart, 2010; Lodeserto, 2018 – Both recommend starting at an FiO_2 of 100% and then dropping down to 40 or 60% to see how the patient does; we can always titrate back up if need be, but if all is well we just leave it there (or even keep titrating down)

ARDS – acute respiratory distress syndrome; **cmH_2O** – centimeters of water; **$EtCO_2$** – end-tidal carbon dioxide; **FiO_2** – fraction of inspired oxygen; **IBW** – ideal body weight; **I-time** – inspiratory time; **kg** – kilogram; **L** – liter; **ml** – milliliter; **min** – minute; **MV** – minute volume

Next step is to look at what extra parameters need to be dialed in on the machine depending on which mode and which control we choose for our patient. As said before, we can ventilate almost any patient in any mode and via any method of control, so long as we know what to monitor for depending on what we choose. And if we are ventilating a patient in pressure control or SIMV (with pressure support), it's OK to just start with the defaults on whatever machine we are working with and then titrate from there given we do so in a timely fashion and with our ventilation goals in mind. Let's draw it all out in another chart:

	additional parameters[173]
Assist Control Volume Control	none
SIMV Volume Control	***pressure support*** – start at 5-10cmH_2O and titrate as needed
Assist Control Pressure Control	***pressure control*** – start at 10-15cmH_2O and titrate to tidal volume goal
SIMV Pressure Control	***pressure control*** – start at 10-15cmH_2O and titrate to tidal volume goal ***pressure support*** – start at 5-10cmH_2O and titrate as needed
Assist Control PRVC	***pressure cap***[174] – set to 25-30cmH_20 (often by setting high-pressure limit to 5cmH_2O above what we want this to be)
SIMV PRVC	***pressure cap*** – set to 25-30cmH_20 (often by setting high-pressure limit to 5cmH_2O above what we want this to be) ***pressure support*** – start at 5-10cmH_2O and titrate as needed

[173] It's a bit tough to identify specific starting points for both pressure control and pressure support in the literature and recommendations vary a lot, but these are points to start off at and then we should always titrate towards exhaled tidal volume and exhaled minute volume goals as soon as possible; as for more insight into these initial settings:
Ashworth & friends, 2018 – They say start with pressure control at 5-10cmH_2O and limit driving pressure (plateau pressure or pressure control minus PEEP, which we will discuss later on **Driving Pressure**) to 16cmH_2O (which correlates with an additive pressure control of that amount)
Kneyber & friends, 2017 – These guys recommend limiting a driving pressure to 10cmH_2O for all (pediatric) patient types
Nagler & Chiefetz, 2019 – This duo suggests a starting pressure support of 5-10cmH_2O for kids
And just to be clear, all the pressures listed here (for pressure control and pressure support) are additive, not cumulative (and for a refresher on what that means, head back to **Types of Breaths**)
[174] Recall that pressure cap is a made-up term and is typically represented by 5cmH_2O less that what we set as the high-pressure limit

OK – alright; **PALS** – pediatric advances life support; **PEEP** – positive end-expiratory pressure; **PRVC** – pressure-regulated volume control; **RR** – respiratory rate; **s** – second; **SIMV** – synchronized intermittent mandatory ventilation; **TV** – tidal volume

At the expense of being overly redundant, let's combine the last two charts into another one to summarize how we determine vent settings, in general and for the normal patient:

step one: set &/ or calculate		**step two: make a choice and dial in extra stuff**	
TV[175]	6-8ml/kg	**Assist Control Volume Control**	none
MV	100ml/kg/min	**SIMV Volume Control**	***pressure support*** – 5-10cmH_2O
RR	adults: 13-17/min kids: use a chart	**Assist Control Pressure Control**	***pressure control*** – 10-15cmH_2O
FiO_2	1.0, then titrate down	**SIMV Pressure Control**	***pressure control*** – 10-15cmH_2O ***pressure support*** – 5-10cmH_2O
PEEP	5-6cmH_2O	**Assist Control PRVC**	***pressure cap*** – set to 25-30cmH_20 (normally: set high-pressure limit to 5cmH_2O above what we want this to be)
I-time	adult: 0.8-1.7s kids: use a chart	**SIMV PRVC**	***pressure cap*** – set to 25-30cmH_20 (normally: set high-pressure limit to 5cmH_2O above what we want this to be) ***pressure support*** – 5-10cmH_2O

In the ideal world, that's how we get vent settings for a specific patient. In the actual world we have a few things to consider (and we'll frame them as questions): What pathophysiologic changes affect the way this patient should be ventilated? What do we do with a patient already being ventilated if settings don't match what we come up with? How does this individual's body respond to all our theoretical stuff? The next few sections will answer these questions in turn. We will first look at specific situations that warrant alterations to this settings framework, then we will talk about setting up the vent in any scenario, and after that we will consider how to evaluate an individual's response to what we are doing with the machine and how we might adjust things to make him or her as happy as possible.

[175] In pressure control we don't actually set tidal volume, but we do need to have a value in mind and calculated out so that we can use it as a goal

ARDS – acute respiratory distress syndrome; **OK** – alright

Specific Vent Strategies

We have a chart from the last section that summarizes the initial calculations and choices we need to make for the average patient and depending on which type of breaths we want to deliver. Next step is to look at exceptions to the norm. To say it another way, sometimes a patient needs his or her breaths delivered in a specific way (different to what we identified as normal) due to intricacies of a given illness or disease. We sometimes take those normal parameters and alter them to meet specific needs and issues. It's totally OK to break the rules we've established so far, as long as we know when and how to do it and can justify a good reason. We will look at a few situations, in turn, to see how it all looks.

Vent strategies are often presented as a choice of two distinct categories: the injured or sick lung approach and an obstructive strategy. We've opted to present this decision-making process as a set of five possible strategies from which providers can choose. This approach is specific to the emergency setting where preventing acute decompensation is a primary concern. First is the general strategy discussed just now, the other four include obstruction, hypotension, acidosis, and lung injury. There is no right or wrong in this process, we just think it makes sense to take things a bit further as we have outlined in the following sections.[176]

---

[176] To provide more context on this two-strategy approach:
The ARDS Network, 2000 – This was a major paper that led the movement towards lower tidal volume with vented patients; while it focuses on a specific patient group (i.e. that injured lung cohort), it set the stage for further research into the idea of much lower tidal volumes than were initially used
Weingart, 2010; Weingart, 2016b – A podcast series and paper, respectively and by the same guy, that outline this two-strategy approach to vent management; while directed towards emergency department physicians, the content is 100% applicable to those of us that work in the transport setting

kg – kilogram; **L** – liter; **min** – minute; **ml** – milliliter; **MV** – minute volume; **OK** – alright; **PEEP** – positive end-expiratory pressure; **RR** – respiratory rate; **s** – second; **TV** – tidal volume

Obstruction

In patients with asthma, COPD, and/ or allergic reaction, we tend to run into a problem of breath stacking or **AutoPEEP** because the patient is unable to exhale fully in a normal amount of time. The pathophysiology is multifaceted and varies a bit depending on underlaying cause, but can be summarized as some combination of the following:

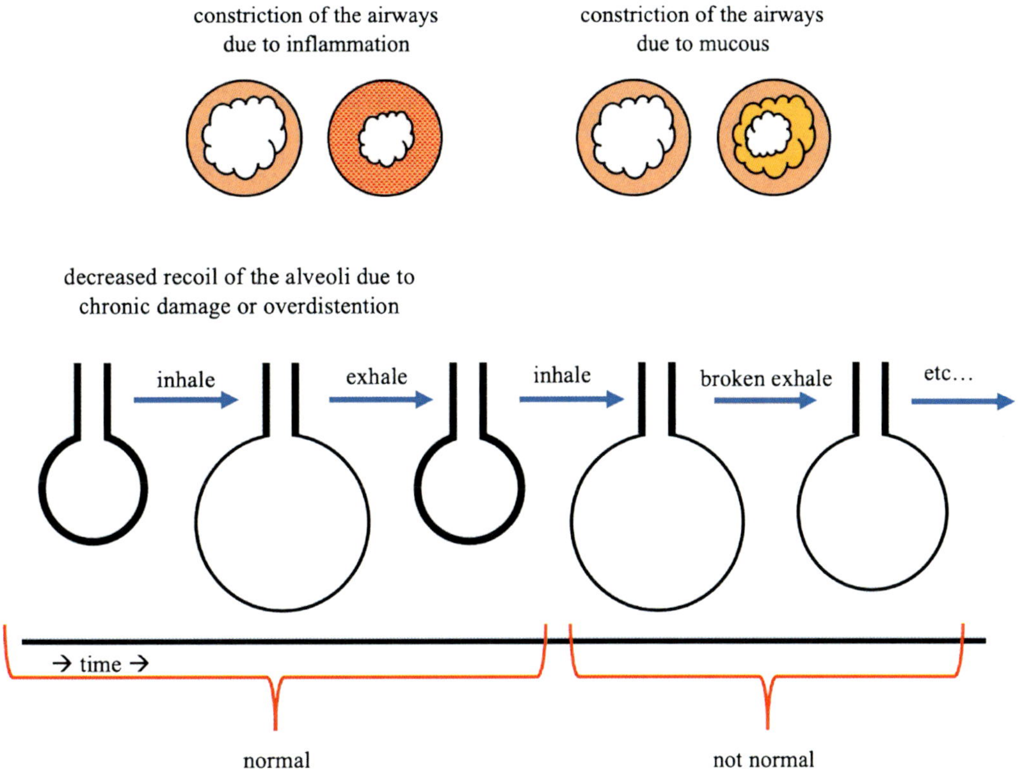

AutoPEEP – intrinsic positive end-expiratory pressure; **cmH₂O** – centimeters of water; **COPD** – chronic obstructive pulmonary disease; **I:E** – inspiratory to expiratory; **I-time** – inspiratory time

The fix is to adjust vent parameters to allow for more time at exhalation. We do this by extending or lengthening the expiratory time (decreasing I:E ratio). A normal I:E ratio is 1:2-3 and we can decrease that by decreasing either the **Inspiratory Time** or **Respiratory Rate**.[177] A good starting point in this population is an I:E ratio of around 1:5. The typical way to get here is to decrease rate (and also inspiratory time) until we see an I:E ratio in that range that we want. The machine normally does this calculation for us, but just an example we'll show it all here:

with I-time 1.0s and RR 17:

$$60 \div 17 \text{ breaths} \approx 3.5\text{s/breath}$$

$$3.5\text{s} - 1.0\text{s (I-time)} = 2.5\text{s}$$

$$\therefore \text{I:E ratio} = 1{:}2.5$$

with I-time 1.0s and RR 13:

$$60 \div 13 \text{ breaths} \approx 4.6\text{s/breath}$$

$$4.6\text{s} - 1.0\text{s (I-time)} = 3.6\text{s}$$

$$\therefore \text{I:E ratio} = 1{:}3.6$$

with I-time 0.8s and RR 13:

$$60 \div 13 \text{ breaths} \approx 4.6\text{s/breath}$$

$$4.6\text{s} - 0.8\text{s (I-time)} = 3.8\text{s}$$

$$\therefore \text{I:E ratio} = \frac{0.8}{0.8} : \frac{3.8}{0.8}$$

$$\text{I:E ratio} = 1{:}4.8$$

So even if we drop both respiratory rate and inspiratory time to the lower ends of our normal parameters, we end up with an I:E ratio shy of what we want for these obstructed patients. Let's keep up with some of these calculations and put them all side by side:

I-time 1.0s		**I-time 0.8s**	
rate	***I:E ratio***	***rate***	***I:E ratio***
17	1:2.5	17	1:3.4
16	1:2.8	16	1:3.7
15	1:3.0	15	1:4.0
14	1:3.3	14	1:4.4
13	1:3.6	13	1:4.8
12	1:4.0	12	1:5.3
11	1:4.5	11	1:5.8
10	1:5.0	10	1:6.5

[177] And as noted back in **Inspiratory Time (and I:E Ratio)**, normal is 1:2 and the 1:3 is more due to convention that what the patient would breathe at if left alone to nature

kg – kilogram; **L** – liter; **min** – minute; **ml** – milliliter; **MV** – minute volume; **OK** – alright; **PEEP** – positive end-expiratory pressure; **RR** – respiratory rate; **s** – second; **TV** – tidal volume

Now let's assume we choose an inspiratory time of 1.0s and a rate of 10 (for a calculated I:E of 1:5.0), what does that do to our other parameters? Biggest thing that will be affected is **Minute Volume**. We'll do some calculations to demonstrate the impact on a 65kg **Ideal Body Weight** patient with a **Tidal Volume** of 8ml/kg:

MV goal = 100ml/kg/min
MV goal = 100ml/kg/min x 65kg
MV goal = 6500ml/min
MV goal = 6.5L/min

TV = 8ml/kg x 65kg
TV = 520ml

MV calculated = TV x RR
MV calculated = 520ml x 10/min
MV calculated = 5200ml/min
MV calculated = 5.2L/min

In fact, we'd have to go up to a tidal volume of 10ml/kg to get to our minute volume goal:

MV goal = TV x RR
6500ml/min = TV x 10/min
TV = 650ml

65kg x ?ml/kg = 650ml
? = 10ml/kg

Now the priority in this strategy for the obstructed patient is to avoid AutoPEEP and allow full exhalation, so start with a focus on rate and I:E ratio. If we need a starting point for tidal volume, just go with the high end of normal or 8ml/kg. Then go down on rate to an I:E ratio of at least 1:5 and monitor for AutoPEEP. After that, we can then titrate up on tidal volume to maintain minute volume as possible. If for some reason we can't go too high on tidal volume due to a high plateau pressure and/ or we have a very low rate due to continued AutoPEEP, minute volume may end up below goal. That's OK in the short term, we just want to try and get as close to it as possible while still allowing for full exhalation and avoiding the AutoPEEP issue.[178] We will simultaneously be doing pharmacologic interventions (Albuterol, Magnesium Sulfate, Ketamine, Epinephrine, whatever our agency endorses) and hopefully the reason for this alternative strategy can get reversed to some degree and then we can go up on rate and work our way back to normal parameters.

[178] Pruitt, 2007; Yartsev, 2019 – The first provides a more in-depth discussion of this permissive hypercapnia approach; the second gives way more information that we thought possible on the potential effects that such an approach may have (but of note, one of those effects may be bronchodilation)

AutoPEEP – intrinsic positive end-expiratory pressure; **cmH_2O** – centimeters of water;
COPD – chronic obstructive pulmonary disease; **I:E** – inspiratory to expiratory; **I-time** – inspiratory time

In **Pressure Control**, we still drop the rate (and maybe inspiratory time too) to lengthen expiratory time (decrease I:E ratio), but we also want as much volume per breath to try and get as close to our minute volume goal as possible. Instead of a pressure control of 10-15cmH_2O, consider going straight to the top and starting at 20-25cm$H_2$0 to see what our exhaled tidal volume values look like.[179] In addition, recognize that this plateau pressure upper limit (30cmH_2O) is a generalization that may not be necessary for all patients.

Second to last thing to mention: it may be tempting to drop **Positive End-Expiratory Pressure** to zero in these cases to better allow the patient to exhale. The thought process goes like so: if they are breathing out while we are pushing air in, this has the potential to be problematic. That said, there is some thought that applied PEEP can help fix AutoPEEP, but we do want to keep applied PEEP lower than AutoPEEP. Just know that we may want to maintain PEEP at our minimum of 5cmH_2O to maximize **Oxygenation** and help recruit more alveoli, but sometimes we let that go in order to avoid AutoPEEP. There may be a happy middle ground with a PEEP somewhere between zero and a normal value, but there isn't much content on that and we'll leave it as a maybe in the overall scheme of things.[180]

Actual last thing to mention: if we have decreased our I:E ratio to accommodate exhalation and we end up at a point where AutoPEEP is consistently zero, we can then titrate our I:E ratio back to normal to make things more comfortable for the patient. This allows us to work back towards our minute volume goal that we started with, as it is likely that our minute volume will be below that goal with a much lower respiratory rate. If things change and obstruction recurs (and then we notice AutoPEEP all over again), we can go back to the smaller I:E ratio (i.e. longer expiratory time). The idea here is that we are constantly reassessing and making these small adjustments to optimize ventilation to the patient in a given moment. Just because a smaller I:E ratio was warranted at the start doesn't mean it is needed forever.

To summarize our obstruction strategy: utilize a lower respiratory rate (and consider a shorter inspiratory time also) to a goal I:E ratio of 1:≥5. Consequently, we need to titrate tidal volume (or pressure control) up as far as the patient's lungs will allow.[181] Know that we will likely be short on our minute volume goal and that's OK. As our pharmacologic interventions start to work we can hopefully migrate back towards normal parameters to meet ventilation goals. Maybe consider dropping PEEP, but know that there isn't yet a good consensus on that. Also, be sure to check for AutoPEEP periodically and consider disconnecting the vent circuit to reset it back to zero if need be.[182]

---

[179] A pressure control value of 25cmH_2O gives us the upper limit for a safe plateau pressure, assuming a PEEP of 5cmH_2O and an additive pressure control value

[180] Stather & Stewart, 2005 – In addition to exploring this idea of using PEEP to mitigate AutoPEEP, these two also provide an overview of a strategy for the asthmatic patient in general

[181] Just remember that it may be harder to get complete exhalation in pressure control ventilation (versus volume control) due to differences in how those breaths are delivered (i.e. decelerating flow versus constant flow, see **Types of Breaths** to review this idea)

[182] We discussed this technique of disconnecting the vent circuit for therapeutic reasons in the section on **AutoPEEP**

min – minute; **ml** – milliliter; **MV** – minute volume; **OK** – alright; **PEEP** – positive end-expiratory pressure; **RR** – respiratory rate; **s** – second; **TV** – tidal volume

Hypotension

In patients with hypotension (or the potential for hypotension) the primary concern is that mechanical ventilation can decrease cardiac output and further contribute to the problem. We discussed this already in reference to both positive-pressure ventilation generally and **Positive End-Expiratory Pressure** specifically.[183] We mentioned then that volume seems to mitigate this effect, so first strategy here (since we are committed to positive-pressure ventilation) is to replace fluids if they aren't contraindicated. Next step is to restrict that PEEP to whatever minimum value we need to maintain adequate oxygenation. Beyond that, we can limit the time spent at inspiration during the overall respiratory cycle. Think of it this way: preload drops further when we increase intrathoracic pressure, so if we decrease the amount of time spent pushing air into the system we can limit this effect.

Now to quantify the idea of how blood return and cardiac output are affected due to breaths given by the machine, consider two patients: one at a **Respiratory Rate** of 17 and one at a rate of 10. If we assume an **Inspiratory Time** of 1.0s (norm for the adult patient), let's calculate how much time the patient experiences a state of decreased preload (i.e. inspiration). We've labeled this idea as percentage of time at decreased preload (%TaDP):

$$\% \text{ TaDP} = (\text{RR x I-time}) \div 60\text{s}$$

with RR of 17

$$\%\text{TaDP} = (17 \times 1.0\text{s}) \div 60\text{s}$$
$$\%\text{TaDP} = 17\text{s} \div 60\text{s}$$
$$\%\text{TaDP} = 28\%$$

with RR of 10

$$\%\text{TaDP} = (10 \times 1.0\text{s}) \div 60\text{s}$$
$$\%\text{TaDP} = 10\text{s} \div 60\text{s}$$
$$\%\text{TaDP} \approx 17\%$$

We can further drop this percentage by decreasing inspiratory time:

with RR of 10 and I-time 0.8s

$$\%\text{TaDP} = (10 \times 0.8\text{s}) \div 60\text{s}$$
$$\%\text{TaDP} = 8\text{s} \div 60\text{s}$$
$$\%\text{TaDP} \approx 13\%$$

[183] See **How is Positive-Pressure Ventilation Different?** to review our discussion on the negative effects of positive-pressure ventilation

%TaDP – percentage of time at decreased preload; **cmH_2O** – centimeters of water; **FiO_2** – fraction of inspired oxygen; **I-time** – inspiratory time; **kg** – kilogram; **L** – liter

By dropping respiratory rate to 10 (from 17) and decreasing inspiratory time to 0.8s (low of normal for the adult patient), we can cut the amount of time at decreased preload by over half. While we could keep dropping respiratory rate, we stop at 10 because we need to maintain minute volume in these patients. Let's look at what happens to **Minute Volume** if we drop the rate to 10 and then come up with a strategy to address it. As before, we'll assume a patient with an **Ideal Body Weight** of 65kg and a **Tidal Volume** of 8ml/kg:

MV goal = 100ml/kg/min
MV goal = 100/ml/kg/min x 65kg
MV goal = 6500ml
MV goal = 6.5L/min

TV = 8ml/kg x 65kg
TV = 520ml
MV calculated = TV x RR
MV calculated = 520ml x 10/min
MV calculated = 5200ml/min
MV calculated = 5.2L/min

Now 5.2L/min isn't super far off from 6.5L/min, but we need to remember that a hypotensive patient is likely at risk of shock and, therefore, we need to make sure that **Ventilation** is adequate by delivering at least what our calculated minute volume minimum is.[184] This idea is in stark contrast to the obstruction strategy in which we decided it was OK to let minute volume fall below goal; in hypotension we need to maintain (or even exceed, especially with **Acidosis** – discussion on that to follow) our minute volume goal. So let's titrate tidal volume up to 10ml/kg and see where we end up:

TV = 10ml/kg x 65kg
TV = 650ml

MV calculated = TV x RR
MV calculated = 650ml x 10/min
MV calculated = 6500ml/min
MV calculated = 6.5L/min

[184] Mannarino, 2014 – Refer to this video for a review of what shock is and how it is related to oxygen delivery

min – minute; **ml** – milliliter; **MV** – minute volume; **OK** – alright; **PEEP** – positive end-expiratory pressure; **RR** – respiratory rate; **s** – second; **TV** – tidal volume

If we drop respiratory rate to 10 (and inspiratory time to low of normal by age) to minimize the percentage of time spent at decreased preload (i.e. inspiration) and increase tidal volume to 10ml/kg, then we maintain our minute volume goal of 100ml/kg/min. Now that we've logically arrived at a strategy of decreased rate and increased tidal volume, let's rewrite the order of the steps as so: increase tidal volume first, then decrease respiratory rate to match minute volume goal. The reason for this is that we don't want to arbitrarily drop respiratory rate and then wind up in a situation where we can't titrate tidal volume up to goal. That would result in a decreased minute volume (which we said is an important thing in the patient at risk for shock). So let's go up on tidal volume as much as we can (even beyond 10ml/kg if we can maintain a safe **Plateau Pressure**) and then drop rate afterward. Even if we aren't able to drop the percentage of time at decreased preload (%TaDP) by half as in the example shown, we can at least move in that direction while ensuring adequate ventilation.[185]

Now there are other justifications for using a high tidal volume and low respiratory rate strategy that don't include this percentage of time at decreased preload (%TaDP) concept, we just find that this makes it easy to appreciate. An alternative justification would be that the strategy decreases dead space.[186] We talked about this idea back when we discussed making changes to address minute volume needs and the idea is that dead space gets introduced with each breath given, so fewer breaths (with more volume each) means less dead space overall.[187] Another rationale would be **Mean Airway Pressure**. This high tidal volume, low respiratory rate approach decreases average pressure into the system, especially when we consider lowering PEEP towards zero (i.e. using the bare minimum necessary to maintain oxygenation). While lowering mean airway pressure could negatively impact **Oxygenation**, we may be able to counteract that with higher FiO_2 to meet our goals. The point here is that there are multiple justifications for this strategy; one has been spelled out here and the other two are deferred until the **Appendix**.

One last thing about this strategy. Similarly to the **Obstruction** approach, if we arrive at a point where we've mitigated the risk of hypotension with adequate resuscitation we can always work back towards normal settings. Even though we put an upper limit on tidal volume by monitoring plateau pressure, recognize that lower values are still preferred for alveolar safety. We'll touch on this again when we get to **Titrating Up on Tidal Volume?**, but realize that if this hypotension strategy is a temporary solution that may not need to be sustained for the entirety of transport or patient interaction.

---

[185] Another advantage of titrating tidal volume first and then rate is that it allows the strategy to be applicable to both adult and pediatric patients without having to come up with more age-based recommendations; while this may or may not be a good reason in and of itself, it does help to keep processes simple and applicable across the board…

[186] Bauer, 2015 – While the strategy discussed in this podcast is slightly different than ours (and includes decreasing PEEP all the way to zero), the basic idea is the same

[187] We discussed this idea of how dead space changes with comparable titrations to respiratory rate and tidal volume back in **Ventilation**

%TaDP – percentage of time at decreased preload; **cmH_2O** – centimeters of water; **FiO_2** – fraction of inspired oxygen; **I-time** – inspiratory time; **kg** – kilogram; **L** – liter

To summarize: in the hypotensive patient we want to decrease the amount of time spent at decreased preload (%TaDP) while maintaining minute volume at our weight-based minimum. To do this, we drop inspiratory time to low of normal, increase tidal volume as much as we safely can manage (in pressure control this may mean starting at 20-25cmH_2O), and then decrease rate to maintain our minute volume goal. We also want to be cautious of high PEEP while recognizing that oxygenation (facilitated by PEEP) is important in these patients with potential low perfusion states. Said one more time in the short and sweet manner of things: when ventilating the hypotensive patient, drop inspiratory, increase tidal volume, drop rate (to maintain minute volume goal), and keep PEEP to a minimum.

Acidosis

We mentioned already that certain factors can impact hemoglobin's affinity for oxygen and pH is one of those things. More acid and lower pH means that oxygen is held less tightly by hemoglobin as it moves through the blood (i.e. hemoglobin's affinity for oxygen is decreased). This makes it more difficult to get oxygen to the tissues where it is needed.[188] While we can increase the amount of oxygen to the alveoli and expect it to diffuse into the blood, getting it from that dissolved state to the hemoglobin itself is the challenge. And then when we do get it loaded onto hemoglobin, it may offload early before getting to the tissues where we intended it to go. To summarize these ideas and a few more, here's how we would draw it all out:[189]

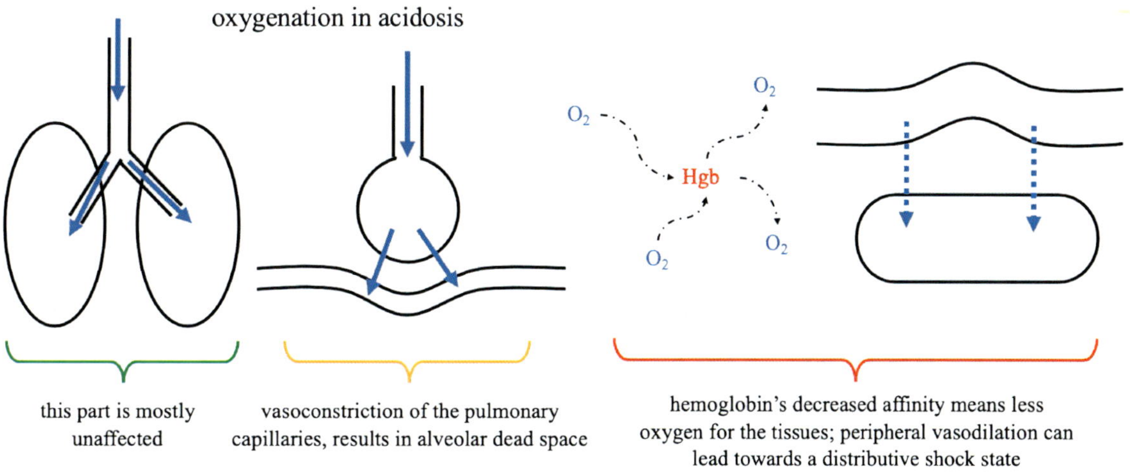

While we still do all the things we already know how to do in regard to **Oxygenation**, the focus of the acidosis strategy we outline here is to work towards correcting these shifts so that oxygen delivery returns to normal. The primary mechanism is to increase **Minute Volume** in an effort to blow off more carbon dioxide. This helps offset the impact of acidosis to some degree. Failing to do so will exacerbate the problem and worsen oxygen delivery with potentially catastrophic consequences.

---

[188] Hasudungan, 2018; Smith, 2014 – The first is a video that reviews this concept of a right shift and also covers some basic physiology we discussed before; the second is a quick video to review acid-base analysis (and for more resources on this, look forward to the section **Patient Already on the Vent**)

[189] Lumb & Slinger, 2015 – Refer back to this article for a review of **Hypoxic Pulmonary Vasoconstriction**

AutoPEEP – intrinsic positive end-expiratory pressure; **$EtCO_2$** – end-tidal carbon dioxide; **Hgb** – hemoglobin; **HCO_3^-** - bicarbonate ion; **kg** – kilogram; **L** – liter; **min** – minute; **ml** – milliliter; **mmHg** – millimeters of mercury

To expand on this, the classic example here is a patient in diabetic ketoacidosis breathing at a **Respiratory Rate** of 30: flight crew comes along, paralyzes and intubates the patient, and then sets the vent up at a "normal" rate of 12. The patient had been compensating with an increased respiratory rate, but that compensation gets taken away suddenly. As a result, the patient quickly decompensates, crashes, and suffers a less-than-ideal outcome.[190] We've already reviewed the idea of oxygenation as it relates to acidosis, but the other factor here is that a rapid increase in $PaCO_2$ can lead to hemodynamic issues such as decreased cardiac contractility, lessened response to catecholamines, and systemic vasodilation.[191] Given all of this, we need a strategy that maintains minute volume both to prevent these hemodynamic effects and to ensure oxygen delivery to the tissues.

While a bit tricky to pinpoint exactly what our minute volume goal ought to be, let's start with a minimum goal double that of the normal patient: 200ml/kg/min.[192] To achieve that goal, we may need to increase both rate and **Tidal Volume**. In order to increase minute volume and get our $EtCO_2$ within a normal range we typically start by changing tidal volume first and then respiratory rate.[193] The reason for this is that adding a breath also adds in dead space to the equation. In the acidosis situation, however, the patient is likely already breathing fast, so let's just use a high of normal tidal volume (i.e. 8ml/kg) and see what kind of rate we'd need to get to this increased minute volume goal of 200ml/kg/min:

$$\text{MV goal} = 200\text{ml/kg/min}$$
$$\text{MV goal} = 200\text{ml/kg/min} \times 65\text{kg}$$
$$\text{MV goal} = 13000\text{ml/min}$$
$$\text{MV goal} = 13\text{L/min}$$

$$\text{TV} = 8\text{ml/kg} \times 65\text{kg}$$
$$\text{TV} = 520\text{ml}$$

$$\text{MV goal} = \text{TV} \times \text{RR}$$
$$13\text{L} = 520\text{ml} \times \text{RR}$$
$$13\text{L}/520\text{ml} = \text{RR}$$
$$25 = \text{RR}$$

---

[190] Weingart, 2009 – And while we don't focus on the intubation process in this manual, look to this throwback episode of EMCrit for a strategy on how to do so while simultaneously avoiding the problems we discuss here

[191] Carter & friends, 2010 – This article focuses how oxygen delivery is affected by acid-base imbalances, but also goes into detail about the consequences of an increased $PaCO_2$ that we mention here

[192] Weingart, 2010 – Our suggestion vaguely resembles the one recommended here (double minute volume to drop carbon dioxide from 40 to 30, that's with a starting minute volume of 120ml/kg/min); that said, this 200ml/kg/min figure is a minimum starting point and we may need to take it further than that – the idea is that we initiate ventilation to prevent immediate deterioration and then go from there to work towards goals (as outlined later in this section)

[193] Deciding which parameter to change (tidal volume versus respiratory rate) to alter minute volume was discussed in **Ventilation**

MV – minute volume; **O_2** – oxygen; **$PaCO_2$** – partial pressure of arterial carbon dioxide; **pH** – power of hydrogen; **RR** – respiratory rate; **SIMV** – synchronized intermittent mandatory ventilation; **TV** – tidal volume

This means that a tidal volume at 8ml/kg and a respiratory rate of about twice normal will get us the theoretical minute volume of 200ml/kg/min. In the normal patient, this would drive our $EtCO_2$ down significantly and create a state of respiratory alkalosis, but we said already that this compensatory respiratory rate is what we want. Now we just need to figure out how to measure or quantify to what extent we are helping the patient. We mentioned in a footnote that this figure (the 200ml/kg/min one) is just a starting point, we then need to be a little more exact in how we go from there. There are a few strategies and we'll talk about them stepwise in order of least exact to more exact.

First thing we can do is to match our rate on the vent to the rate at which the patient was breathing before we took that respiratory effort away. This assumes that the patient was compensating adequately beforehand and that we are the ones intubating or taking that airway away. And while this doesn't give us a quantitative goal to work towards, it is better than nothing. We can match the patient's effort with our settings and then simply monitor for changes. Or if we can do gasses en route, we can always start this strategy and then evaluate progress along the way.

Another strategy is to measure the patient's $EtCO_2$ prior to taking the airway. We can do this via a side-stream nasal canula device or by using an in-line $EtCO_2$ device with non-invasive ventilation.[194] We can then match the patient's respiratory rate (as above) or set the rate to twice normal and then adjust to this $EtCO_2$ that the patient was at before we messed with things. Again, this strategy is similar to the above strategy in that it requires that the patient was compensating adequately on his or her own before we intervened.

A third approach is to utilize Winter's Formula to establish an $EtCO_2$ goal. The formula looks like so:

$$PaCO_2 = (1.5 \text{ x } HCO_3^-) + 8 \pm 2$$

The formula is designed to measure the respiratory component with a known metabolic acidosis (i.e. measured $PaCO_2$ is compared to a calculated $PaCO_2$ to determine if the patient is compensating adequately or if a mixed disorder is present),[195] but we can modify its use in the transport setting to guide our titration of EtCO2 (via minute volume).[196] This strategy is of use if we are taking over care of an acidotic patient who is already on the ventilator:

$$EtCO_2 \text{ should be } \leq (1.5 \text{ x } HCO_3^-) + 8$$

[194] Weingart, 2009 – We referenced this podcast already on the previous page, but take a look for a step-by-step discussion of this strategy for intubating the acidotic patient while maintaining minute volume in the preoxygenation phase with non-invasive positive-pressure ventilation

[195] Foster & Grasso, 2014 – Short video to explains Winter's Formula and its normal use in a clinical setting

[196] Lodeserto, 2018 – See *Part 3* of this series, it gives another perspective on how to manage the vented patient with concurrent (severe) metabolic acidosis; part of that discussion is another formula by which we can quantify a desired minute volume to achieve a $PaCO_2$ goal – we've left that part out here, but it is worth taking a look

AutoPEEP – intrinsic positive end-expiratory pressure; **$EtCO_2$** – end-tidal carbon dioxide; **Hgb** – hemoglobin; **HCO_3^-** - bicarbonate ion; **kg** – kilogram; **L** – liter; **min** – minute; **ml** – milliliter; **mmHg** – millimeters of mercury

A few notes about all of this: $EtCO_2$ generally correlates with $PaCO_2$ fairly well, with $EtCO_2$ normally 2-5mmHg below $PaCO_2$. That normal difference is due to anatomic dead space and will increase with additional dead space (i.e. alveolar dead space). That said, even with more dead space in play, $EtCO_2$ and $PaCO_2$ will move in stepwise fashion at the same rate.[197] If we use this modified formula, adjust minute volume to that goal, and get our $EtCO_2$ right at the calculated value based on HCO_3^- from labs, we still may be a bit shy of our minute volume goal. Just keep that in mind and know that's why we wrote it out as we did without the "±" and with the "≤." If it helps, think of this value we get from the modified Winter's Formula as an upper limit for $EtCO_2$ in the patient with metabolic acidosis.

One more point to make is that the HCO_3^- can be from either the metabolic panel or arterial blood gas for our use in the transport setting, but know that there are varying opinions on that.[198] Regardless of source, however, it is best if the HCO_3^- is from a current set of labs. The longer it has been since the been since that value was initially obtained, the less applicable that value becomes to the current situation. In the event that the most recent HCO_3^- is more than a few hours in the past and that no prior data exists on pre-intubation respiratory rate or $EtCO_2$, the situation becomes a little less clear. We could still aim for that minute volume goal of 200ml/kg/min and use the Winter's Formula approach, especially in cases where the patient's ventilation has not been maintained at these goals since labs were measured. We may also consider decreasing sedation to allow the patient to better express a need for more minute volume and evaluate things subjectively. We could even make it easier for the patient to trigger breaths by titrating our trigger threshold.

To bring it all home, we can do all of these strategies together: try to match the patient's respiratory rate and $EtCO_2$ as measured before intervention, then compare both minute volume to our calculated minimum goal of 200ml/kg/min and $EtCO_2$ to a goal derived from Winter's Formula. And if we aren't the ones taking the airway and intubating, the Winter's Formula approach is likely the best strategy. If that isn't an option, however, we may be able to let the patient guide treatment by decreasing sedation and trigger thresholds and allowing the patient to take the lead. The only next best thing here would be to measure gasses en route to see how the patient is responding to treatment, but most of us don't have that capability in the field and we'll withhold a discussion of it here.

---

[197] Siobal, 2016 – And look here for more information on carbon dioxide monitoring in general

[198] Nargis & friends, 2015 – This is because in the metabolic panel it is a measured quantity, in the arterial blood gas it is calculated and there can be some discrepancy between the two values; all that said, there is strong correlation between the two and it likely doesn't much matter in the majority of cases; and while this particular study was looking at the totally unrelated idea of cost-effectiveness related to blood gas analyzers in the developing world, the findings on correlation between the two values are still worthwhile

MV – minute volume; **O_2** – oxygen; **$PaCO_2$** – partial pressure of arterial carbon dioxide; **pH** – power of hydrogen; **RR** – respiratory rate; **SIMV** – synchronized intermittent mandatory ventilation; **TV** – tidal volume

One more thing to mention in regard to modes: because we are shooting for a high minute volume in the acidotic patient, **Assist Control** may be the best for these patients if they are triggering breaths. If we do go **Synchronized Intermittent Mandatory Ventilation** and the patient has spontaneous effort to breathe, consider increasing pressure support so that patient-triggered breaths match machine-delivered ones (and this would avoid a drop in minute volume if we were following the normal SIMV strategy of pressure support breaths below tidal volume goal).[199] In either case, the idea is to match the patient's need for more minute volume as expressed by effort to trigger more breaths. As always, monitor airway pressures and be sure that **AutoPEEP** is not an issue. We definitely don't want to get in a situation where minute volume drops due to the development of AutoPEEP and the cycling off of breaths due to our high-pressure alarm.[200]

We went on a bit of a tangent here, but let's get back to our vent strategy for the acidotic patient: use a tidal volume goal high of normal (8ml/kg) and increase rate (either to match patient's intrinsic rate or even just double normal for patient's age), then aim for a goal minute volume of 200ml/kg/min and an $EtCO_2$ of patient's baseline prior to intervention or as determined by Winter's Formula. The goal of the acidosis strategy is to maintain minute volume in order to prevent oxygen delivery from getting worse, to work towards correcting the underlaying imbalance, and to prevent any acute decompensation from a rapid rise in $PaCO_2$.

---

[199] We talked about this idea that pressure support breaths are often smaller than the time-triggered or mandatory ones way back in the section on **Synchronized Intermittent Mandatory Ventilation**; also review **Assist Control** mode

[200] We discussed this idea of dropping minute volume due to AutoPEEP and the high-pressure limit back already, but will do so again when we get to **Alarms**

4x4 – four-by-four dressing; **ARDS** – acute respiratory distress syndrome; **AutoPEEP** – intrinsic positive end-expiratory pressure; **CO_2** – carbon dioxide; **cmH_2O** – centimeters of water; **$EtCO_2$** – end-tidal carbon dioxide; **FiO_2** – fraction of inspired oxygen

Lung Injury

Another much-discussed strategy in vent management is the injured or sick lung strategy, also known as the lung-protective approach. This is for patients that have lungs particularly susceptible to further injury and barotrauma and, as a result, we use less volume per breath in an effort to avoid over-inflation. We then have to increase **Respiratory Rate** to maintain **Minute Volume** or be OK with an elevated $EtCO_2$. Another component of this strategy is higher than normal **Positive End-Expiratory Pressure**, which helps via a few different mechanisms. We'll start by reviewing the concept of acute lung injury and discussing the pathophysiology of acute respiratory distress syndrome, then we'll get into specifics about vent strategy.

Acute lung injury (ALI) refers to a number of pathologies that inhibit normal pulmonary gas exchange.[201] Specific causes include sepsis, pneumonia, bleeding from a traumatic injury, inhalation of toxins or smoke, and aspiration. Acute lung injury is a concept that lives on a spectrum with acute respiratory distress syndrome (ARDS) being the most severe endpoint. While acute lung injury, as a term, may also be described as mild or moderate ARDS, the underlying pathophysiology is the same. The main component of the disease process is that the alveolar and capillary walls become permeable to stuff that is normally sequestered in the blood:

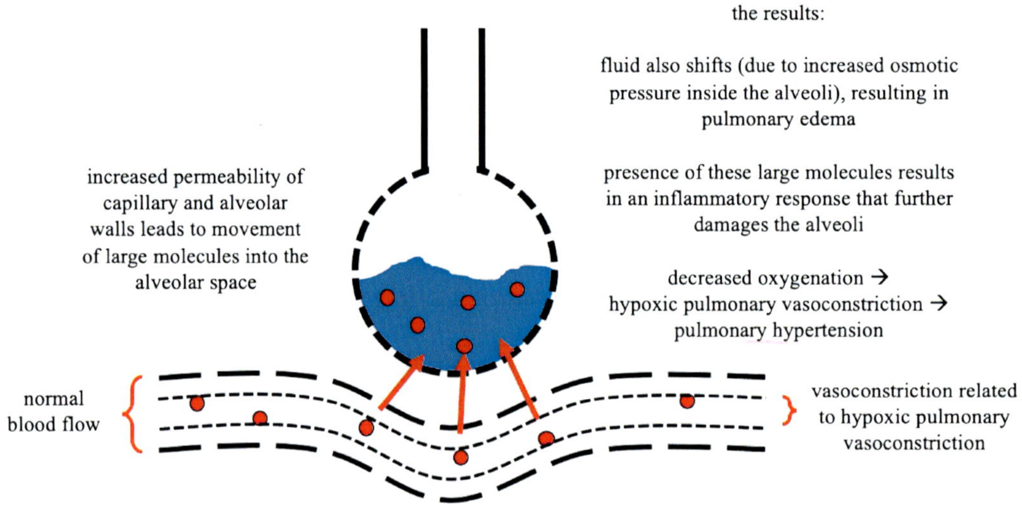

[201] Ragaller & Richter, 2010 – Not only do they provide an overview of the acute lung injury/ ARDS disease process, they also discuss this whole vent strategy and summarize research to date (at least as of 2010)

kg – kilogram; **L** – liter; **min** – minute; **ml** – milliliter; **mmHg** – millimeters of mercury; **MV** – minute volume; **OK** – alright; **PaO₂** – partial pressure of arterial oxygen; **PEEP** – positive end-expiratory pressure; **RR** – respiratory rate; **SpO₂** – pulse oximetry; **TV** – tidal volume

There are quantitative criteria for acute lung injury and/ or ARDS (depending on how we choose to define it), but that isn't necessary for our field treatment. Given our capabilities in the transport setting, we generally identify a patient who needs this vent strategy from a report per sending facility or suspicion based on clinical progression of the illness. There are also many recommendations to use this strategy for all patients who don't fit any other category.[202] In this sense we could think of the lung injury approach as we outline it here as a general strategy. We'll come back to that idea at the end of this section, but for now let's move on to the details. As we noted at the start, this lung injury strategy includes low **Tidal Volume**, higher than normal PEEP, and a focus on recruitment. Let's discuss each of these in turn and give some specific guidance.

Starting tidal volume for these patients should be 6ml/kg **Ideal Body Weight**, but we may get as low at 4ml/kg eventually. This recommendation is from a classic ARDSNet study which compared a tidal volume of 6ml/kg to 12ml/kg and determined that lower tidal volume resulted in better outcomes for these patients.[203] While it may seem that 6ml/kg and 12ml/kg represent two extremes and it could be tempting to rationalize that 8 or 10ml/kg probably isn't all that bad, we do know that 6ml/kg is OK and the rest is still up to debate at this point.[204]

---

[202] And in the case of two-strategy recommendations, it is either this lung injury approach or an **Obstruction** strategy that make up the choices

[203] The ARDS Network, 2000 – Much of the data we have on contemporary vent management comes from this group of researchers and subsequent investigations by other folks based on their research

[204] Sahetya & friends, 2017; Burrell, 2018 – And for a more detailed discussion of this, take a look at this article (summarizes different arguments for why tidal volume ought to be tightly controlled in ARDS) and that review of another paper (which sought to investigate this idea of using a tidal volume in that middle area between 6ml/kg and 12ml/kg)

4x4 – four-by-four dressing; **ARDS** – acute respiratory distress syndrome; **AutoPEEP** – intrinsic positive end-expiratory pressure; **CO_2** – carbon dioxide; **cmH_2O** – centimeters of water; **$EtCO_2$** – end-tidal carbon dioxide; **FiO_2** – fraction of inspired oxygen

In addition to low tidal volume, we go up on PEEP to improve both **Oxygenation** and **Ventilation**. As previously discussed, PEEP facilitates oxygenation by increasing **Alveolar Surface Area**, moving fluid out of the alveoli, and facilitating gas exchange through the expiratory side of the breath cycle. As for ventilation, PEEP actually helps to reduce **Dead Space** allowing for less wasted ventilation and better clearance of carbon dioxide.[205] Just know that this effect is limited and that PEEP taken too far can actually contribute to more dead space. Also recognize that when titrating PEEP, smaller changes with more time in between are less damaging to the alveoli and we likely won't be able to fix these patients in the time we spend with them during transport (i.e. don't get overly aggressive with increasing pressure over a short amount of time). And last thing, consider titrating PEEP alongside FiO_2 in a stepwise fashion as outlined in the charts below:[206]

OXYGENATION GOAL: PaO_2 55-80 mmHg or SpO_2 88-95%
Use a minimum PEEP of 5 cm H_2O. Consider use of incremental FiO_2/PEEP combinations such as shown below (not required) to achieve goal.

Lower PEEP/higher FiO2

FiO_2	0.3	0.4	0.4	0.5	0.5	0.6	0.7	0.7
PEEP	5	5	8	8	10	10	10	12

FiO_2	0.7	0.8	0.9	0.9	0.9	1.0
PEEP	14	14	14	16	18	18-24

Higher PEEP/lower FiO2

FiO_2	0.3	0.3	0.3	0.3	0.3	0.4	0.4	0.5
PEEP	5	8	10	12	14	14	16	16

FiO_2	0.5	0.5-0.8	0.8	0.9	1.0	1.0
PEEP	18	20	22	22	22	24

[205] Robertson, 2015; Murias & friends, 2014 – PEEP can help reduce dead space, but only up to a certain point; after that PEEP actually contributes more to the problem

[206] NHLBI ARDS Network, 2005 (image); NHLBI ARDS Network, 2004 – The study cited shows that either of those two approaches is appropriate; in fact, they modified the study in process to test even higher PEEP – we've left that out just to keep things a little simpler, but also because there is ongoing debate as to whether or not PEEP is the best strategy by which to improve outcomes in these patients

kg – kilogram; **L** – liter; **min** – minute; **ml** – milliliter; **mmHg** – millimeters of mercury; **MV** – minute volume; **OK** – alright; **PaO_2** – partial pressure of arterial oxygen; **PEEP** – positive end-expiratory pressure; **RR** – respiratory rate; **SpO_2** – pulse oximetry; **TV** – tidal volume

Another really important component of our lung injury strategy is alveolar recruitment. This is a concept that we've talked about some, but we'll get into it more here.[207] Recruitment is the idea that we can actively re-inflate collapsed or underinflated alveoli as we drew out in our previous discussion of PEEP. One component of the acute lung injury/ARDS disease process is that the alveoli are particularly susceptible to both barotrauma and stress due to repetitive expansion and collapse. By slowly filling the alveoli with air and then using small volumes of air with each breath, we maximize usable space within the lungs and avoid causing damage. PEEP allows us to make this happen (i.e. it maintains recruitment through this process) and in turn we may have to sacrifice net movement of air per a permissive hypercapnic approach (i.e. we sacrifice some degree of ventilation to maximize oxygenation).

A few things about all of this: incomplete oxygenation in the ARDS patient is often due to ventilation/ perfusion (V/Q) mismatch and under-perfused regions of lung.[208] We previously said that our parameters to improve oxygenation are **Fraction of Inspired Oxygen**, **Positive End-Expiratory Pressure**, and **Inspiratory Time**. Even if we have all of these things optimized, we may still be short of our oxygenation goals and that's just part of the disease process. Further fixes for that ventilation/ perfusion (V/Q) mismatch would include time (i.e. being patient), minimizing dead space, and maintaining adequate ventilation.[209] While we often hear ARDS strategies described with a component of permissive hypercapnia, that idea is questioned by some and may go contrary to our overall goals. There are varying opinions on this, however, so initiate a dialogue with sending or receiving facilities if specific questions about management of these patients becomes an issue.

Getting back on track with the idea of recruitment, if we have alveoli stented open with PEEP and then disconnect the vent circuit, those alveoli go back to a baseline, deflated state. In a normal lung there are forces that maintain recruitment to prevent this loss and we can also re-recruit alveoli on the order of seconds to minutes. This means that for the normal patient it isn't a huge deal for us to be worried about losing recruitment. We just get them on the vent again, add a bit of PEEP, and we are back where we want to be with no real negative outcome. With the lung injury patient, however, it can take hours to recruit alveoli. If we lose recruitment with these patients, we lose all of that progress towards better oxygenation and ventilation, and our patient can deteriorate very quickly.

[207] And then we will talk about recruitment again when we get to **Recruitment Maneuvers**

[208] Radermacher & friends, 2017 – This paper goes into lots of detail on how the gas exchange process is affected in ARDS and how treatments have changed over time as new evidence emerges

[209] To review these ideas: we talked about both the time factor and how alveolar dead space can be caused by ventilation/ perfusion (V/Q) mismatch in **Hypoxic Pulmonary Vasoconstriction**; we discussed **Dead Space** previously in that section and then again just a moment ago when we mentioned that PEEP can help to reduce dead space

With that in mind, it is important to keep the system that extends from the vent to the patient's alveoli intact at all times. When we do have to break the system, such as when we transfer the patient from our machine to the hospital's machine or vice versa, we can maintain recruitment by clamping off the endotracheal tube. The point is to prevent pressure at the alveoli from dropping below PEEP. While it theoretically doesn't matter at which point in the respiratory cycle we clamp the tube and perform the swap, just to be safe let's do this clamping of the tube during inspiration. That way, we have a cushion of safety if we leak some air out in the process. And here is what the technique looks like:

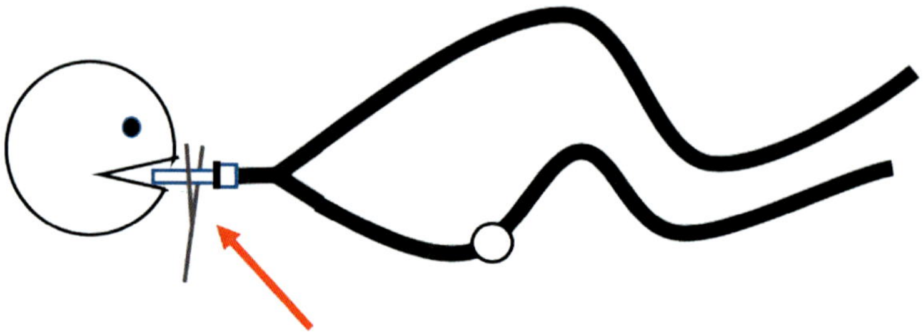

clamp endotracheal tube with hemostats before disconnecting (consider using a 4x4 to pad things so that the teeth on the hemostat don't damage the tube)

Last thing to mention with this lung injury strategy is minute volume. We mentioned already that we start at a tidal volume of 6ml/kg and may need to go down to 4ml/kg. With higher PEEP we increase overall airway pressures and therefore that 6ml/kg tidal volume on top of a higher PEEP (up to 20 in some cases) means we might run into a high **Plateau Pressure**. If we notice plateau pressure encroaching on our safe limit of $30cmH_2O$, then we can dial the tidal volume down to 5ml/kg and then to 4ml/kg (or if we are in pressure control we can just go up on PEEP and look at exhaled tidal volume). Dropping our tidal volume to 4ml/kg will reduce minute volume and increase $EtCO_2$, but let's quantify that difference in minute volume with an assumed patient of 65kg ideal body weight:

MV goal = 6.5L

TV = 4ml/kg x 65kg
TV = 260ml

MV calculated = TV x RR
MV calculated = 260ml x 17/min
MV calculated = 4420ml
MV calculated ≈ 4.4L

kg – kilogram; **L** – liter; **min** – minute; **ml** – milliliter; **mmHg** – millimeters of mercury; **MV** – minute volume; **OK** – alright; **PaO_2** – partial pressure of arterial oxygen; **PEEP** – positive end-expiratory pressure; **RR** – respiratory rate; **SpO_2** – pulse oximetry; **TV** – tidal volume

And to maintain our MV goal, let's see what kind of RR we would need:

$$\text{MV goal} = \text{TV} \times \text{RR}$$
$$6.5\text{L} = 250\text{ml} \times \text{RR}$$
$$6.5\text{L} / 250\text{ml} = \text{RR}$$
$$25 = \text{RR}$$

So to maintain our minute volume goal with a tidal volume of 4ml/kg we need a respiratory rate of 25 for the adult patient. With pediatrics (when a rate of 25 is too slow), we just go up on respiratory rate as much as we can to meet (or exceed if in volume control) our minute volume goal. Consider doubling respiratory rate, or using the high end of normal for a given age range, or just titrate up from a normal rate. The limiting factor will be comfort and exhalation (i.e. monitor for AutoPEEP to ensure full exhalation).[210] And as we mentioned just a moment ago, there is some evidence that permissive hypercapnia (i.e. a high $EtCO_2$ related to a lower minute volume) is alright for these lung injury patients, but the data isn't super clear at this point.[211]

To put it all together: lung injury represents a spectrum of disease that primarily impacts the integrity of the alveolar and capillary walls; this results in increased permeability, movement of large molecules and fluid into the alveolar space, and further damage from an inflammatory response. Vent strategy is focused on low tidal volume starting at 6ml/kg (down to 4ml/kg if needed) to avoid barotrauma, high PEEP to both maintain recruitment of alveoli and displace fluid, maintenance of recruitment at all transfers in order to avoid rapid deterioration, and an increase in rate to maintain minute volume (possibly with a concurrent strategy of permissive hypercapnia).

And one last thing to mention about this strategy. We said just a moment ago that lots of folks recommend a two-strategy approach to ventilation in which we use either this lung injury approach or an obstruction approach. We have a general vent strategy for routine ventilation and then specific strategies for certain patient types. The differences between our general strategy (which is similar to a general lung-protective one) and this lung injury strategy is related to recruitment of alveoli (both using high PEEP and being super careful to not lose it) and the idea that we may need to go down on tidal volume to 4ml/kg. Both of these things are totally OK in the normal patient that we ventilate using the general strategy, it's primarily a matter of emphasis. If it makes things easier to default to this lung injury strategy in all cases that don't warrant one of the others, that's completely acceptable.

---

[210] A few notes on this: we talked about this overshooting of minute volume in the section on **Volume Control** and will do so again in the **Appendix**, also, the likelihood of transporting a pediatric patient with ARDS is slim and low-frequency, so ask for help and/ or consult with a specialist on this

[211] Just to clarify: the idea here is that permissive hypercapnia is tolerable for the lung injury patients, not that it provides an extra benefit

COPD – chronic obstructive pulmonary disease; **cmH₂O** – centimeters of water; **EtCO₂** – end-tidal carbon dioxide

Other Potential Strategies

This list of vent strategies addresses four markedly different situations that we often come across in the transport setting, but there are other injuries or disease processes that might also warrant specific adjustments to the normal list of settings. While we could theoretically compile a list of all the possible things and work out an algorithm to address each one in turn, that gets a little cumbersome and would result in a hefty protocol that might be difficult to navigate through when time is of the essence. The idea is to work towards an understanding of how the body responds and how the vent does its thing so that we can make changes and anticipate the results that will come of any adjustment away from normal. But just to mention a few examples without going into the same level of detail as we did just now, consider the following situations.

In the patient with a head injury or traumatic brain injury, we often choose to aim for an $EtCO_2$ low-of-normal to what we'd typically use for a standard patient.[212] While we don't necessarily hyperventilate these patients anymore, we could adjust **Minute Volume** to a tighter $EtCO_2$ goal of 35-40mmHg by going up on either **Tidal Volume** (preferred) or **Respiratory Rate**. Carrying on with this idea: we want to simultaneously avoid hypoxic events and minimize the effects of too much oxygen. We also want to find a balance between maintaining comfort to avoid increases in intracranial pressure and being able to perform neuro assessments to track patient progress. All that said, consider using tighter parameters and/ or reassessing these patients more often.[213]

In the pregnant patient we might utilize a **Fraction of Inspired Oxygen** of 100% to maximize oxygen delivery to the fetus. Since many services don't have the capability of fetal monitoring during transport, this is a way to ensure that we don't have a hypoxic injury or put any undue stress on the fetus. We also need to consider an increased minute volume goal for the patient (which may mean an $EtCO_2$ goal low of normal, somewhere in the 30-35mmHg range), as we have a baby to consider as well.[214] Another consideration is patient positioning. In the vented pregnant patient we not only have decreased preload due to positive-pressure ventilation, we could see that drop in cardiac output compounded by pressure of the fetus on the inferior vena cava. So either turn the patient to a lateral recumbent position or displace the gravid uterus over to the side.

Significant chest trauma is another one. We'd like to treat these patients via the **Lung Injury** strategy, but we may also be concerned with hemodynamics and want to use the **Hypotension** strategy. Those two are at odds with one another (low tidal volume and high respiratory rate for lung injury, high tidal volume and low respiratory rate for hypotension). Maybe we forgo the hypotensive strategy and choose the lung injury one, but get aggressive early on with vasopressors and fluids and/ or blood products in anticipation that a hypotensive state may be precipitated by our strategy. Or maybe we go with a strategy more in line with the hypotensive strategy, but start with lower **Positive End-Expiratory Pressure** and leave FiO_2 at 100%. There is no right or wrong here and it depends a lot on how the patient presents in that particular situation and what resources we have to work with.

---

[212] Godoy & friends, 2017 – Detailed overview of ventilatory management in traumatic brain injury with a review of research that has been done to date

[213] Refer back to **Oxygenation** for a discussion of the negative effects of oxygen and then to **Comfort** for a review of strategies to work towards ventilator synchrony

[214] Wingfield, 2012a; LoMauro & Aliverti, 2015 – The idea of a lower $EtCO_2$ goal with the pregnant patient is suggested in a video by the first guy; the physiology behind it is discussed in an article by the other two

FiO_2 – fraction of inspired oxygen; **mmHg** – millimeters of mercury; **OK** – alright; **PEEP** – positive end-expiratory pressure

On a tangent to this chest trauma idea: if a patient develops a tension pneumothorax en route, the best thing we can do may be to take the patient off the vent.[215] Not take them off the vent and bag them, but take them off the vent and don't breathe at all for them until we fix that problem. Positive-pressure ventilation can tension a pneumothorax very quickly and we want to avoid making things worse.[216] While this is more of an issue with pneumothorax caused by acute trauma and it isn't unheard of to see patients in a relatively stable condition while vented with a pneumothorax in the hospital, in transport we will likely notice a pneumothorax after it has started to tension and that is a true emergency. So disconnect the vent, decompress (or place a chest tube/ perform a finger thoracotomy), and then get the patient back on the vent. Because of this, we may consider keeping all patients with the potential for pneumothorax on a FiO_2 of 100%. That allows us more time to perform the procedure, if a pneumothorax develops, before the patient desaturates.

A patient with congestive heart failure or pulmonary edema may warrant more PEEP to facilitate the movement of fluid out of the alveoli.[217] In addition, PEEP might help drop afterload to facilitate both perfusion and clearing of fluid from the pulmonary side of circulation. And while it may make sense that a high FiO_2 could mitigate the effects of an **Hypoxic Pulmonary Vasoconstriction** effect in these patients, there is some risk to that strategy and treatment focused on adequate minute volume and PEEP are preferred with congestive heart failure.[218] Folks with chronic obstructive pulmonary disease may ought to have oxygenation tightly controlled due to the potential effects of oxygen.[219] We could even argue the case for a specific toxic-exposure strategy: some combo of lung injury plus or minus **Acidosis**, depending on the agent and route of exposure.

It quickly becomes evident that there are a number of cases that don't quite fit the mold by which we try to simplify vent strategies. And that's totally OK. The templates are there as frameworks from which we then consider the specifics of each patient, one at a time. The important thing is to know what impact any vent change will have on the patient depending on how (s)he presents in a given situation. There are lots of cases in which there isn't a straightforward answer, but as long we don't make things worse by titrating things the wrong way, all is good.

---

[215] Flowers & friends, 2019 – Per Boyle's Law (increase in volume with a decrease in pressure), we can cause this tension by taking a stable pneumothorax to elevation

[216] Wingfield, 2012b; Hsu & Sun, 2014 – Both of these sources discuss pneumothorax in the mechanically ventilated patient; the first discusses this idea of removing these patients from the vent immediately, the second is an overview of the idea and outlines a simple algorithm for managing these patients

[217] Perlman & friends, 2010 – While a plateau pressure up to $30cmH_2O$ is likely still just fine with these patients, just know that pulmonary edema can make the patient more susceptible to injury (and the authors outline why that might be via a unique experiment)

[218] Kuhn & friends, 2016 – This article reviews mechanical ventilation strategies for patient with heart failure; while it focuses on the extreme end of these patients (i.e. decompensated heart failure), some of the ideas could apply to congestive heart failure patients on a general sense

[219] Swaminathan, 2015 – Short discussion of oxygen administration in COPD with a focus on investigating some of the common misconceptions

AutoPEEP – intrinsic positive end-expiratory pressure; **cmH_2O** – centimeters of water; **LPM** – liters per minute

Additional Concepts, Round One

Before we get to putting these various strategies into action, there are just a few more concepts to cover. We've touched on some of these in passing already, but let's take the time to look at them in a bit more detail so we are better prepared when it comes time to lay everything out in a plan of action.

Triggers

Triggers are the thresholds by which the machine knows when a patient is trying to breathe on his or her own. We first tried to communicate this idea via the following graphic:

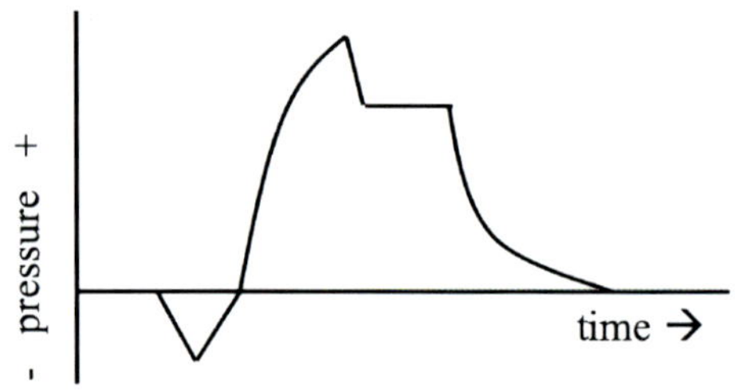

And then we footnoted the idea that that downward dip in pressure at the start of the waveform is more a sketch of convenience than an accurate representation of how things normally occur.[220] In most cases the trigger that makes the machine recognize patient effort is based on flow rather than pressure. While some machines will allow us to use pressure triggers (normally around $-1cmH_2O$), this isn't commonly used. Pressure triggers have been shown to be more difficult for patients to overcome (at least with older model ventilators). In addition, the pressure trigger is relative to what we have dialed in for **Positive End-Expiratory Pressure**. This means that in the event of **AutoPEEP** there is an extra threshold that must be overcome:

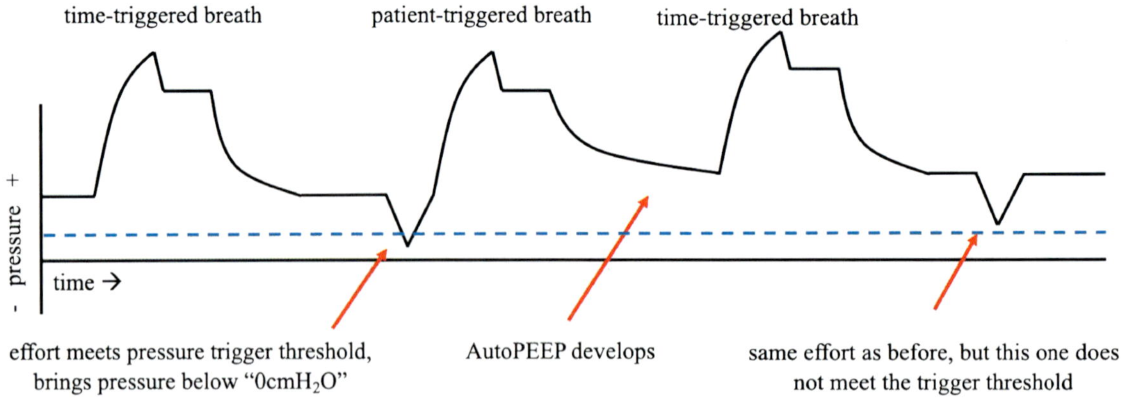

[220] We first drew this waveform out when we were talking about **Modes of Ventilation**, specifically the section on **Assist Control**

So pressure triggers are a thing as we initially drew it out, but not the most common thing. We sometimes do use pressure triggers in cases of auto-triggering (i.e. when we see too many triggered breaths due to things other than patient effort, such as bumpy roads in an ambulance or turbulence in an aircraft), but for the most part we stick with flow triggers.[221] To measure flow changes against a zero reference (the pause between breaths is a zero-flow state) the machine uses a concept called bias flow. Bias flow is a baseline flow of air into the system against which changes are measured. So when the machine says there is no flow going into the system, there is actually some flow going in, but it gets factored out. Let's draw it out with an assumed bias flow of 5LPM just to see how it works:[222]

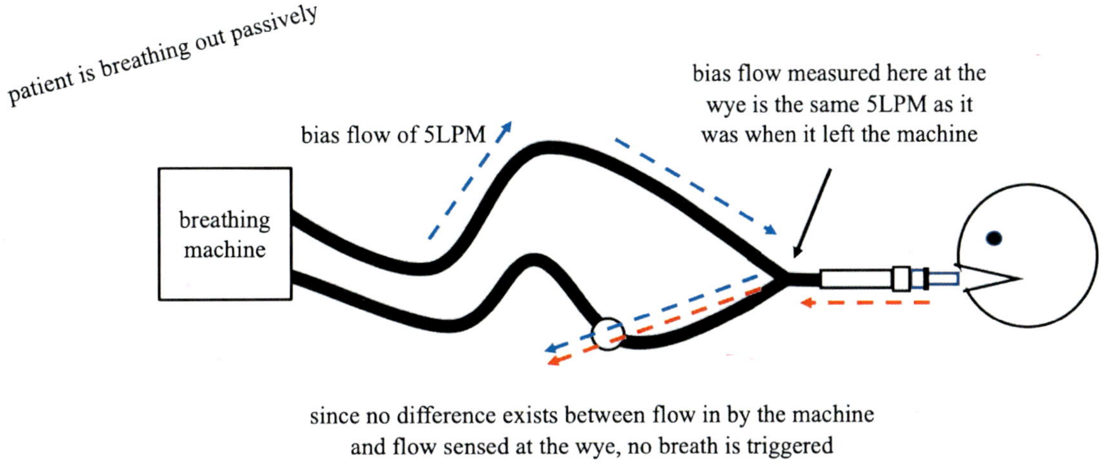

[221] Hess, 2005 – While we could utilize pressure triggers to mitigate worsening AutoPEEP with increased patient respiratory effort (assuming an initial flow trigger), we prefer to address the cause of discomfort or meet the patient's demands rather than ignoring it altogether

[222] Yartsev, 2019 – For an alternative explanation of how this flow trigger works (plus much more detail on triggers in general), take a look at this article

AutoPEEP – intrinsic positive end-expiratory pressure; **cmH₂O** – centimeters of water; **LPM** – liters per minute

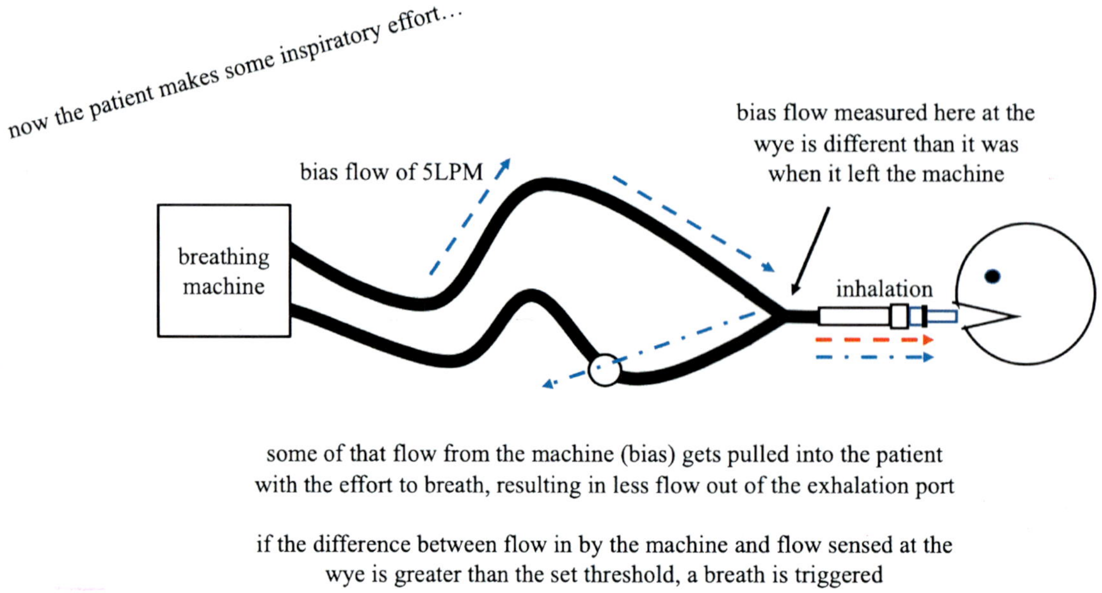

The machine does this bias flow thing because it makes it easier to measure patient effort. Bias flow can either be set manually or adjusted automatically by the machine based on what we have set as the flow trigger.[223] It's not something we routinely consider in transport, but if we are working with a machine in which bias flow is manually controlled it's worth knowing that we can't have a trigger set higher than our bias flow. So if our machine has a bias flow of 5LPM and we want a trigger higher than that, we would have to increase the bias flow.

A normal flow trigger in the hospital setting is 1-2LPM. This value is also referred to as sensitivity (i.e. a sensitivity of 2LPM would indicate a flow trigger of 2LPM). For reference, the normal mean flow produced by a human at rest is about 15LPM with a peak of about twice that.[224] Which means we could theoretically dial our flow trigger much higher than the 1-2LPM that we normally use and still expect a patient to trigger breaths. As we discussed previously, we titrate sensitivity to allow patient effort to trigger breaths, but also to prevent other miscellaneous input from accidentally causing triggers.

---

223 Chatburn & Mireles-Cabodevila, 2013 – For a brief discussion of bias flow, scroll down to *The Operator Interface* and then *Flow* within this chapter

224 Yartsev, 2019 – We cited this website on the last page, but he specifically outlines the norms for both in-hospital flow triggers and flow produced by normal respiration which we cite here

AutoPEEP – intrinsic positive end-expiratory pressure; **cmH_2O** – centimeters of water; **LPM** – liters per minute

To expand on this idea, let's consider things sequentially. If breaths are being triggered, first thing is to try and identify what input is causing the triggers. If it seems likely that the input is patient effort, all is well. If, however, there is something else that is causing the trigger (i.e. auto-triggering), then we troubleshoot that. Bumpy roads or turbulence (especially with the vent circuit laying on the floor of the vehicle) and accidentally kicking or stepping on the circuit are common causes of auto-triggering. The preferred approach is to fix those things directly and solve the problem without changing the sensitivity on the machine. If, however, we cannot alleviate the accidental triggering of breaths, then we can increase the trigger sensitivity or consider a different type of trigger (i.e. change from a flow trigger to a pressure trigger). The idea is to simultaneously prevent breaths from being accidentally triggered and keep the trigger threshold as low as possible so that it is easier for the patient to meet the trigger.

To summarize triggering: triggers are thresholds we set to allow the machine to know that the patient wants to take a breath. We most commonly use flow triggers, but some machines allow for pressure triggers as well. Flow triggers are based on and limited by bias flow. A sensitivity of 1-2LPM is commonly used in a hospital setting. Auto-triggering happens when the trigger is inadvertently met by something other than patient effort to breathe. Fixes to auto-triggering include mitigating the cause of the inadvertent trigger, increasing the sensitivity, or trialing a different type of trigger.

$EtCO_2$ – end-tidal carbon dioxide; **I:E** – inspiratory to expiratory; **$PaCO_2$** – partial pressure of arterial carbon dioxide

Overbreathing

Just to close the loop on one idea that we mentioned back in the section on **Vent Parameters, Round One**, let's consider what to do if we think the patient is breathing too fast and/ or in a way that goes contrary to how we want to manage **Ventilation**. Say we have a patient breathing faster than we'd like and, as a result, our $EtCO_2$ is low. Normally we'd decrease **Respiratory Rate** to drop **Minute Volume** and get that $EtCO_2$ back in range, but now we have to consider these patient-triggered breaths and the fact that decreasing the parameter on the vent won't decrease the overall rate. First thing to think about is that an increased rate of breathing is the body's normal response to lots of things: decreased pH or increased $PaCO_2$ (as we discussed in **Acidosis**), pain, fluid in the lungs, irritants in the airways, anemia, cardiac ischemia, etc.[225] So before we label this overbreathing as an anomaly and decide that something needs to be done, consider that it may actually be an appropriate response.

On a tangent to this idea, if the concern is minute volume in a general sense and not necessarily respiratory rate, we can simply decrease **Tidal Volume** or consider switching from **Assist Control** to **Synchronized Intermittent Mandatory Ventilation** to try and bring minute volume down. It's important to remember that minute volume is the product of both respiratory rate and tidal volume. Even though we routinely modify respiratory rate to address an excessive minute volume, decreasing tidal volume is also an appropriate strategy. But if we don't have an identifiable cause and rate is the thing we want to fix, the next considerations to address too many patient-triggered breaths are **Comfort** and **Triggers**. We talked already about both of these ideas, so we won't get into too much detail here. The general idea is that if patient-triggered breaths are the issue (i.e. too many of them happening), we can fix that by either reducing discomfort, manipulating the trigger threshold itself, and/ or avoiding accidental triggers.

There is one more thing to note about this. We mentioned back in **Basic Modes of Ventilation** that both controlled mechanical ventilation and intermittent mandatory ventilation are modes that do not have a mechanism for patient-triggered breaths. We said then that some ventilators allow us to approximate these modes (i.e. ignore patient effort to breathe) and theoretically that would be an option in the case of overbreathing. That said, this strategy is likely to be very uncomfortable for the patient and would probably require heavy sedation and maybe even paralysis to work. We generally don't want to simply ignore patient efforts, rather we would prefer to do things to promote synchrony and work alongside the patient.

Back to our discussion, if we've ruled out all of these situations and the patient is still breathing too fast and we've already considered both comfort and triggers, what else is there to do? First thing is to verify that the increased respiratory rate (the cumulative total of our set rate plus patient-triggered breaths) is, in fact, a problem. It may be the case that the patient is breathing fast, but with no identifiable negative outcome. Reassess the patient with a focus on the **Three Big Things** and then decide if it's still a problem that needs to be addressed. If so, we have a few options: **Positive End-Expiratory Pressure**, increasing tidal volume, and paralytics.

---

[225] Murphy, 2017a; Alexander, 2016 – The first is one video of three part series on control of breathing, feel free to check out the others for more; the second is an article about tachypnea in general, provides some insight on overlooked causes of tachypnea

PEEP – positive end-expiratory pressure; **pH** – power of hydrogen

Adding PEEP can be more comfortable for a patient (which may lead to fewer triggered breaths) and will also reduce minute volume while keeping the lungs open and participatory in ventilation. Just recognize that in **Volume Control** ventilation we will need to reevaluate pressures to ensure that the alveoli remain safe (i.e. that our **Plateau Pressure** is still acceptable). Moving forward, there is also the idea that increasing tidal volume can lead to less dyspnea or air hunger due to an effect on chemoreceptors in the lungs.[226] And then if we increase tidal volume and exceed the minute volume needs of the patient, they will respond will a slower rate of breathing. While this is a bit counterintuitive, it could be worth trialing. And at the extreme end of things we could administer paralytics, but we prefer to reserve that strategy for life-threatening situations.

As a related example, let's say we have a ventilated patient who suddenly experiences acute bronchospasm or has an anaphylactic reaction. Per our **Obstruction** strategy we would like to decrease our I:E ratio by decreasing both **Inspiratory Time** and **Respiratory Rate**. So we do that on the vent, but the patient is still triggering breaths for an actual or calculated I:E ratio higher than we'd like and with the result that **AutoPEEP** starts to develop. At this point the rate dial on our machine is not the primary way we control the overall rate and we need to think about other ways to bring the patient's intrinsic rate down to achieve our goals. Similar to what we said above, strategies here would include further decreasing inspiratory time, addressing comfort, making sure triggers are appropriate, and adding PEEP.

So while we've discussed adjusting respiratory rate up to this point as if it were a parameter we have complete control over via the machine interface, recognize that the number of breaths per minute can exceed the value we have set. Patient-triggered breaths are generally of benefit to the patient, but if they threaten overall wellbeing or safety then we ought to take action to get things back on track.[227] Steps to fix this problem include addressing comfort, evaluating triggers, adding PEEP, trailing an increased tidal volume, and, as a last resort, paralysis.

[226] Banzett & friends, 2013 – For a very detailed discussed of this idea, take a look at this chapter in Tobin's textbook on vent management

[227] This idea that patient-triggered breaths can be of benefit was discussed back in the section on **Comfort**

ΔP – driving pressure; **ΔV** – change in volume; **ARDS** – acute respiratory distress syndrome; **AutoPEEP** – intrinsic positive end-expiratory pressure; **cmH_2O** – centimeters of water; **LPM** – liters per minute

Driving Pressure[228]

Driving pressure (ΔP) is a term to describe how much we inflate and deflate the alveoli with every inhale and exhale on the ventilator. The idea is that too much opening and closing (inflation and deflation, up and down – however we want to term it) can put stress on the alveolar walls and cause damage.[229] This damage, in turn, leads to decreased diffusion of gasses across the alveolar membrane. Driving pressure is the difference between **Plateau Pressure** and end-expiratory pressure (normally **Positive End-Expiratory Pressure**, but sometimes affected by **AutoPEEP**) and is also referred to as delta pressure:

$$\Delta P = Pplat - PEEP$$

As an image, it would look like this:

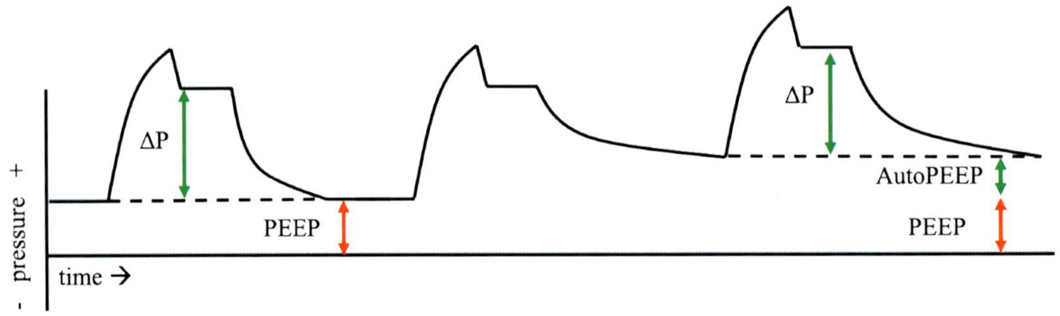

With our **Lung Injury** patients, we try to limit driving pressure as much as we can to a max of $15cmH_2O$.[230] This is generally pretty reasonable, given that we use high PEEP and low **Tidal Volume** in these patients anyways. And if driving pressure is close to or above that upper limit, we can do **Recruitment Maneuvers** to try and utilize more lung, increase compliance, and drop driving pressure.[231] This approach may sound familiar and is often referred to as open-lung ventilation.[232] The basic idea is that we keep the lungs as filled as possible (i.e. alveoli inflated) throughout as much of the respiratory cycle as we can. This concept of limiting driving pressure and an open-lung strategy is specific to the ARDS population.

---

228 Bugedo & friends, 2017 – Succinct overview of the concept of driving pressure and research done to date (as of a few years ago, at least)

229 Grune & friends, 2019 – While it is commonly accepted that this inflation/ deflation cycle does cause damage (and we will assume it to be valid in our discussion), know that there is ongoing research on all of this (as shown in this article)

230 Weingart, 2016a; Bauer, 2016b – Both podcasts look at a 2015 study on the subject of driving pressure

231 We will discuss **Compliance (and Resistance)** and **Recruitment Maneuvers** in the next two sections

232 Nickson, 2019b – We will get much more into this idea of open-lung ventilation shortly, but this page provides a nice overview of the concept to hold us over until then

ml – milliliter; **PEEP** – positive end-expiratory pressure; **PIP** – peak inspiratory pressure; **Pplat** – plateau pressure; **TV** – tidal volume; **VTe** – exhaled tidal volume

With that said, there may be the case for a comparable strategy in other patient groups, there just hasn't been much research on that to date. The one downside of this limited driving pressure or open-lung approach is that it can be tough to blow off carbon dioxide as much as we'd want.[233] We said way back when that permissive hypercapnia is often a thing with ARDS, but that may not be the case with other patient groups. Another consideration here is PEEP – it is not a benign thing and we for sure need to consider the negative consequences of this approach before applying it to all patients. For now we have pretty good evidence that limiting driving pressure and utilizing high PEEP is a good thing with ARDS, but such a strategy may not be best for everyone.

Compliance (and Resistance)[234]

Compliance is a measure of how much the lungs fill per unit of pressure put into the system. In math terms it looks like this:[235]

$$\text{compliance} = \frac{\Delta V}{\Delta P} = \frac{\text{TV or Vte}}{(\text{Pplat} - \text{PEEP})}$$

While normal compliance (healthy and breathing spontaneously) is somewhere in the neighborhood of 100ml/cmH_2O, we often see values much smaller than that in our ventilated patients. The best way to utilize compliance during transport is to keep track of trends: increasing compliance is good, decreasing compliance is bad. If we do something that results in poorer compliance, maybe second guess whatever that change was; if we do something that results in better compliance, high fives are warranted. Acute causes of decreased compliance would be a worsening pneumothorax, inhibition of chest wall expansion, chest wall rigidity caused by certain medications, increasing **Tidal Volume** beyond the capacity of the lungs at that given time, etc.[236]

---

[233] To say it another way: by limiting driving pressure, **Ventilation** may be affected and **Minute Volume** may be less than we might want

[234] Trainor & friends, 2019 – This video reviews both compliance and resistance in a succinct and straightforward way

[235] To be more specific, this is what we would call static compliance; we won't get into dynamic compliance here

[236] All of these high **Peak Inspiratory Pressure**, high **Plateau Pressure** situations will be discussed in the section on **Watching Pressures**

ΔP – driving pressure; **ΔV** – change in volume; **ARDS** – acute respiratory distress syndrome; **AutoPEEP** – intrinsic positive end-expiratory pressure; **cmH_2O** – centimeters of water; **LPM** – liters per minute

A related term is resistance. Resistance and compliance are often discussed together under the umbrella terms of respiratory mechanics or pulmonary mechanics, that's why we talk about it here.[237] Now the algebraic expression of resistance isn't quite as straight forward as for compliance and we often simplify it by assuming that flow equals 60LPM, so we're just going to skip on ahead and note it like this:

$$\text{resistance} = \text{PIP} - \text{Pplat}$$

Resistance, in this simplified manner, is the limitation to air movement that must be overcome for us to arrive at a state in which air in from the machine gets to the alveoli. Assuming plateau pressure remains constant, resistance is represented by peak inspiratory pressure. This means that we can approximate changes to peak inspiratory pressure to signify changes to resistance. So things like kinks in the tubing, biting on the tube, excessive secretions, etc. that are causes of increased peak pressure and unchanged plateau pressure correlate with an increase in resistance:[238]

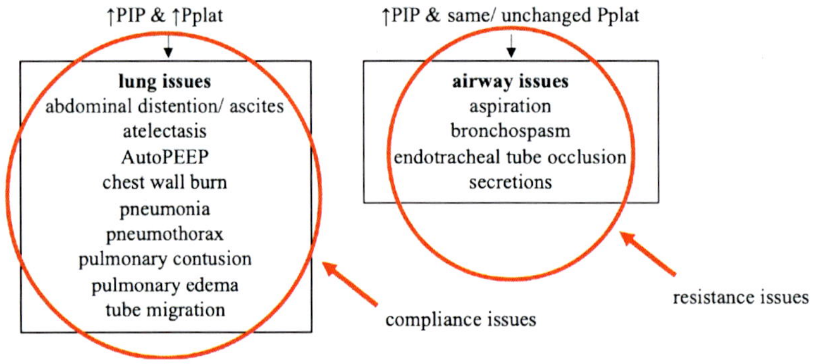

And we mentioned already that the alternative strategy in **Pressure Control** ventilation when we don't have peak inspiratory pressure or plateau pressure to guide us is to look at exhaled tidal volume and exhaled minute volume to gauge when these things are happening (a drop in volume will indicate an increase in resistance or decrease in compliance). We can also look at a quantitative value for compliance (if available to us on our machine) or see how flow is changing from breath to breath.[239]

---

[237] Hess, 2014 – And for much more on this concept of respiratory mechanics and all the other things included, refer to this guide
[238] Cassone & friends, 2019 – We will expand on this in **Watching Pressures**, but know for now that this graphic is a piece of an algorithm that we lay out when we get there – it just made sense to include it here to differentiate these two concepts
[239] Again, this in pressure control only; in volume control flow will be the same with each breath delivered

mmHg – millimeters of mercury; **O_2** – oxygen; **PEEP** – positive end-expiratory pressure; **PO_2** – partial pressure of oxygen; s – second; **SpO_2** – pulse oximetry

Recruitment Maneuvers

A recruitment maneuver is a technique that attempts to get more alveoli involved in the breathing process.[240] During ventilation, and even at health, there are portions of the lung that are open or participatory and others that are closed down or non-participatory (or maybe just less-than-optimally-participatory), and we can do things to gain access to those clamped-down alveoli to improve both **Oxygenation** and **Ventilation**:

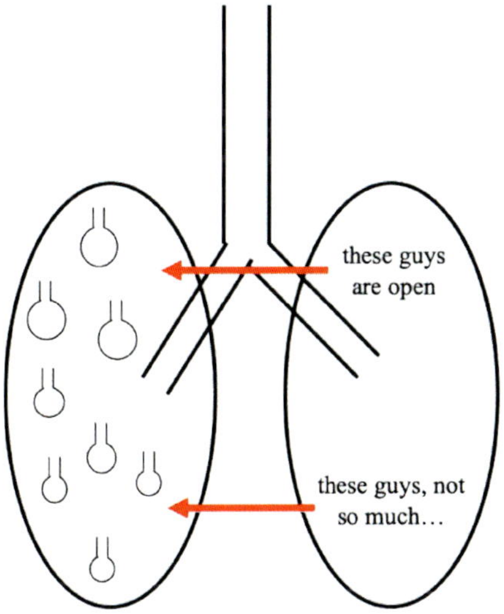

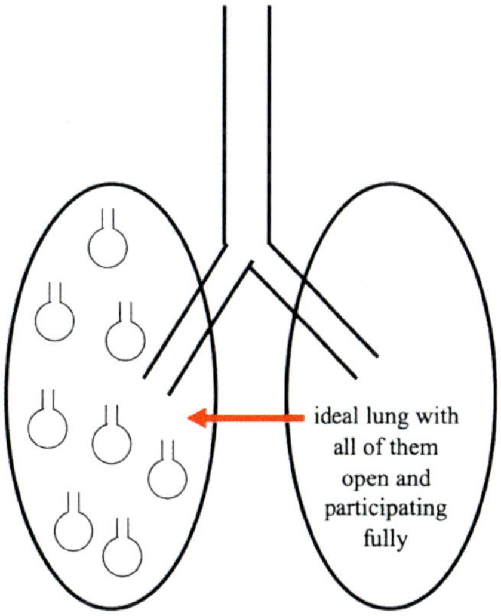

In a general sense, lots of things could qualify as recruitment maneuvers: prolonged inspiratory holds, higher **Positive End-Expiratory Pressure**, high-frequency oscillation ventilation (HFOV),[241] airway pressure release ventilation (APRV),[242] **Prone Ventilation**, spontaneous breathing, etc. Basically anything that can help open those non-participatory alveoli falls into this category.[243] That said, we tend to consider recruitment maneuvers to be either the prolonged inspiratory hold or the stepwise approach, so we will stick with those two ideas moving forward.[244]

---

[240] Ragaller & Richter, 2010 – We talked about the advantages of getting more alveoli involved in the breathing process both in **Alveolar Surface Area** and **Oxygenation**; the article is an overview of ARDS management with a section on the idea of recruitment; it also refers to the idea of open-lung ventilation, which we will discuss momentarily

[241] Prost, 2011 – This is the only mention we have of HFOV, as it isn't routinely available in transport; the referenced video is an overview of it

[242] Farkas, 2017 – While APRV isn't common in transport at the moment, chances are we will start to see more of it in years to come; navigate here for a discussion of this mode in the context of an open-lung approach (discussed on the next page); also refer to many more references at the bottom of the page

[243] Naik & friends, 2015 – This is an article that also discusses recruitment, but particularly the idea that breaths of various sizes (whether intentional via vent management or spontaneous via patient effort) further contribute to recruitment

[244] Hartland & friends, 2015 – This paper both discusses recruitment maneuvers and describes their use in non-ARDS patients under anesthesia

APRV – airway pressure release ventilation; **ARDS** – acute respiratory distress syndrome; **cmH_2O** – centimeters of water; **HFOV** – high-frequency oscillation ventilation

A recruitment maneuver can be used in any patient group, but has been most studied with ARDS patients under the umbrella term open-lung ventilation. We can think of open-lung ventilation as a supplement to the lung-protective approach we described in **Lung Injury**. The focus of lung protection is smaller **Tidal Volume** and keeping **Plateau Pressure** within normal limits. The open-lung idea adds to that a component of utilizing recruitment maneuvers to get more alveoli involved.[245] While these two ideas (lung-protective and open-lung) are not universally defined and there is some overlap, the general idea hold true.

Recruitment maneuvers have been shown to increase oxygenation and improve ventilation/ perfusion (V/Q) mismatch, but outcomes in terms of mortality and days on the vent seem to be unaffected or even worse.[246] To further complicate things, when we do try and get into the weeds as to how we should perform a recruitment maneuver, techniques vary significantly and there are potential adverse effects. So here's where we stand on this: more data is clearly needed, but there is low-quality evidence that some benefit exists from performing recruitment maneuvers in ARDS patients, particularly as part of an overall open-lung strategy.[247] Translating that to the non-ARDS patients who are simply hypoxic is a bit tough, as there isn't much data out there and we can often fix the issue by way of things we've already talked about (**Fraction of Inspired Oxygen**, **Positive End-Expiratory Pressure**, and **Inspiratory Time**) and ensuring adequate perfusion.[248]

But let's say we do want to do a recruitment maneuver anyways. Maybe we are struggling to oxygenate a patient, or we forgot to clamp the endotracheal tube on transfer of an ARDS patient to our vent, or we want to try for better **Compliance** and/ or decreased **Driving Pressure**, etc. First thing to know is that the maneuver can cause hemodynamic problems and we ought to be on the lookout for those to avoid decompensation. Just as we discussed back when we first got into **How is Positive-Pressure Ventilation Different?** and PEEP, an increase in intrathoracic pressure can drop preload and subsequently impact cardiac output. So monitor all the things and have hard limits in place for abandoning the maneuver.[249] Also, recognize the risk for causing a tension pneumothorax and consider that an underinflated tube cuff or uncuffed pediatric tube will render the maneuver less effective.[250]

---

[245] Nickson, 2019b – Refer here for an outline-style overview of this open-lung strategy and its components

[246] van der Zee & Gommers, 2019 – This article describes much of the research that has gone into understanding recruitment maneuvers, particularly in the context of an open-lung approach

[247] Hodgson & friends, 2016 – Cochrane Review that summarizes the data on recruitment maneuvers in ARDS

[248] These steps were discussed in **Oxygenation**

[249] Claire & friends, 2019 – And for suggestions on limits to use while performing one of these maneuvers and an explanation of the next technique (the stepwise recruitment maneuver), take a look at this short guide

[250] Chambers & friends, 2017 – This study primarily examined how exhaled tidal volume differed from delivered tidal volume with cuffed and uncuffed tubes, but it also looked at the effect recruitment maneuvers have on this difference

mmHg – millimeters of mercury; **O_2** – oxygen; **PEEP** – positive end-expiratory pressure; **PO_2** – partial pressure of oxygen; **s** – second; **SpO_2** – pulse oximetry

The simplest way to do a recruitment maneuver is via a prolonged inspiratory hold.[251] We posed a hypothetical situation at some point earlier on in this manual about why we don't just blow up the lungs and alveoli with oxygen and let it sit like that for a while. We said then that we still have to consider the ventilation side of things, but the idea itself does have some merit. The value of a recruitment maneuver (again, this is as a prolonged inspiratory hold) is more in the ability to get alveoli open than in the inflow of oxygen for a sustained amount of time, as the amount of oxygen in that air quickly begins to drop as it diffuses into the bloodstream and we don't replenish the supply:

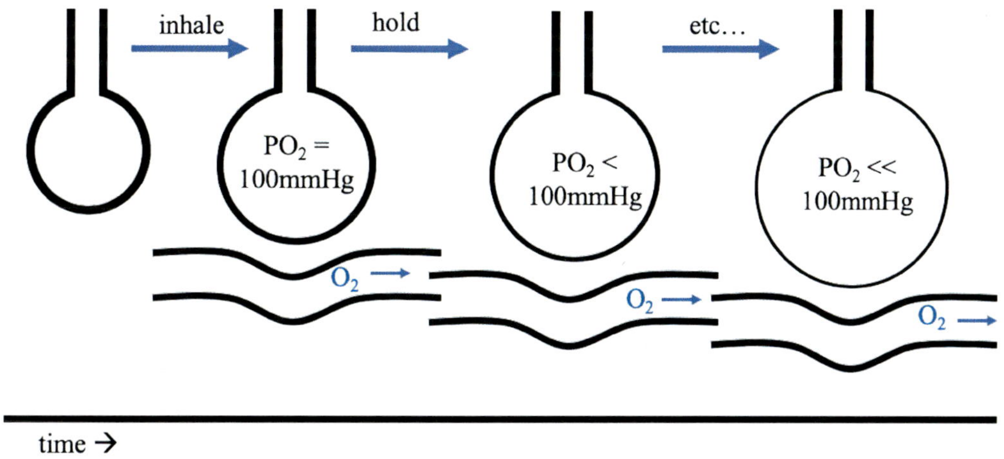

To perform a prolonged inspiratory hold as a recruitment maneuver, here's how it works: Put the patient in **Pressure Control**, set the pressure control parameter to achieve a goal pressure (keeping in mind that we may or may not need to factor PEEP into this), and perform an inspiratory hold for as long as we deem appropriate. Recommendations on specifics vary widely, but a pressure of 30-40cmH_2O for about 30s is often cited.[252] That said, there are many opinions that a hold beyond ten seconds doesn't provide any additional benefit.[253] There's also the question of how often we ought to or can perform these maneuvers. Most of the data out there is specific to in-patient settings with these maneuvers performed relatively infrequently, so this isn't something that would perform many times throughout transport, rather we may do it once after getting a patient set up on our vent.[254] We won't get into specifics beyond that, as this would be a better conversation to have with both the providers involved in a specific patient case and medical direction within a given agency.

---

[251] Metz, 2016a – Video that shows a prolonged inspiratory hold in a set of lungs attached to a vent circuit

[252] NHLBI ARDS Network, 2004; Hartland & friends, 2015 – While a few other references cited in this section also mention a prolonged inspiratory hold in line with these two articles, it seemed appropriate to note some things: this type of maneuver was tested by the ARDSNet folks and subsequently discontinued during the trial; the other study used a similar maneuver plus two others and found positive benefit with any of them prior to patients undergoing surgery

[253] Radermacher & friends, 2017 – Knowing that a prolonged inspiratory hold may not have benefit beyond ten seconds and given the fact that performing the maneuver in general can affect hemodynamics means we should probably limit the length of these types of recruitment maneuvers

[254] Hodgson & friends, 2016 – While this review doesn't directly outline a specific frequency at which recruitment maneuvers should be performed, it does allude to the idea that they are done intermittently throughout a (hospital) shift or once per day

APRV – airway pressure release ventilation; **ARDS** – acute respiratory distress syndrome; **cmH₂O** – centimeters of water; **HFOV** – high-frequency oscillation ventilation

Moving on to the next type of recruitment maneuver, we have the stepwise approach. We mentioned already that whenever we put more air into the lungs it seems advantageous to do so incrementally. Same goes for performing a recruitment maneuver. An alternative to the prolonged inspiratory hold would be a stepwise approach.[255] In **Volume Control** we would simply increase PEEP incrementally and over time; in pressure control we would establish a driving pressure that yields our goal tidal volume, then slowly titrate up on PEEP in in a similar fashion.[256] There is a rendition of this approach called the Staircase Recruitment Maneuver that seeks to identify the point of maximal benefit by observing SpO_2 as PEEP is titrated back down from the point of maximum pressure.[257] This is particularly important to keep in mind, as the benefit of a recruitment maneuver (i.e. the involvement of more alveoli) may not be sustained if we subsequently revert back to a PEEP that we were at before the maneuver.

In any event, the utility of recruitment maneuvers is to get more alveoli involved in ventilation. This improves compliance and allows us to ventilate to our tidal volume goal with lower driving pressure while working to correct ventilation/ perfusion (V/Q) mismatch across the lung and improve oxygenation.[258] While there are risks involved and the data is a bit vague when it comes to long-term benefits, it seems fair to conclude that if we mitigate those risks by using a stepwise approach and monitoring for patient decompensation along the way there is likely some use in the transport setting.

---

[255] Metz, 2016b – Another video showing a version of the stepwise recruitment maneuver on a set of lungs attached to a vent circuit
[256] Hess, 2015 – This paper outlines these types of stepwise recruitment maneuvers and has a graphic to show how they increase usable volume in the lungs over time
[257] Claire & friends, 2019 – See this page for a step-by-step description of how to perform the Staircase Recruitment Maneuver
[258] Hartland & friends, 2015 – We cited this study back when we discussed absorption atelectasis in **Oxygenation**; while it looks at a specific group of patients we don't often encounter in transport (those undergoing abdominal surgery), the findings support the idea than recruitment maneuvers are of benefit in the short term (which is likely comparable to the transport setting)

I:E – inspiratory to expiratory; **kPa** – kilopascal; **mmHg** – millimeters of mercury; **OK** – alright

Make a (Calculated and Informed) Plan

This next section covers how we go about setting the patient up on the ventilator. In particular, it looks at how the process differs when it's us initiating ventilation versus if we are taking over a patient in which ventilation has already been initiated. This may not seem like a big deal, but the taking over of a vented patient is a bit tricky. Even though we have these predetermined strategies for different patient types, the truth is that there is a lot of variation in how patients respond to the vent. Sometimes an asthmatic patient is happy with an I:E ratio of 1:2, other times a hypotensive patient has a high respiratory rate and low tidal volume for good reason, etc. Because of this, we need a method to determine when changes are needed and when we can leave things alone as we find them.

Getting the Intel Ready

The first thing we do for any patient who needs to be or is already ventilated is to listen. We listen to a report from whoever was hanging out with the patient before we got there. This is very important for all patients, as it can tell us how the patient has responded to or will respond to strategies we might have in mind. We then (as in *after* listening) decide on a strategy based on how we think that patient ought to be ventilated. Next we get an accurate patient height (either from a reliable healthcare provider or by measuring it ourselves) and perform three calculations: **Ideal Body Weight**, **Tidal Volume**, **Minute Volume**.

Following that is the patient exam. We'll discuss a few of the specifics when we talk about a patient already on the vent, but we for sure want to get an exam done before we start manipulating things or playing with our vent. Our mental construct of a strategy based on the report we received should match what we see in the exam. If not, we need to clarify that amongst ourselves before moving forward. No need to elaborate on that here, we all know the importance of a good assessment. So once we have a report, have done an assessment, and are decided on a strategy, we move forward.

From Scratch

When we are the ones initiating the vent, it's fairly straightforward: we take the settings we've come up with based on presentation and pathophysiology, then plug them into whatever mode and method of control we decide to use. We've already talked about the different strategies and why we may choose to use one mode or control over another, so we won't spend any more time on that here. The easiest way to do this is to stick with whatever our machine defaults to and then adjust from there if need be. Once the patient is on the ventilator, we just need to confirm that everything is going as planned, beginning with the **Three Big Things**: oxygenation, ventilation, and comfort. Once we get those things sorted, we can then move on to some of the finer subjects (which will be discussed in the next section, **Keeping Things Going**).

Just to reiterate: the settings we conceptualize prior to initiating ventilation (and as discussed in the previous sections) are starting points from which we then make adjustments. It may very well turn out that we end up with settings, based on patient need, that vary significantly from what we initially had in mind and that's OK. But the starting point ought to be based on an understanding of what is going on with the patient and calculated goals. And if we have no idea which strategy to choose or if the patient fits too many categories all at once, just start with those basic settings we discussed in **A General Vent Strategy** and go from there.

AutoPEEP – intrinsic positive end-expiratory pressure; **$EtCO_2$** – end-tidal carbon dioxide

Patient Already on the Vent

With someone already on the vent, it gets a little more complicated. We'll draw it out in a short, simple algorithm first and then we will expand on it as we go:

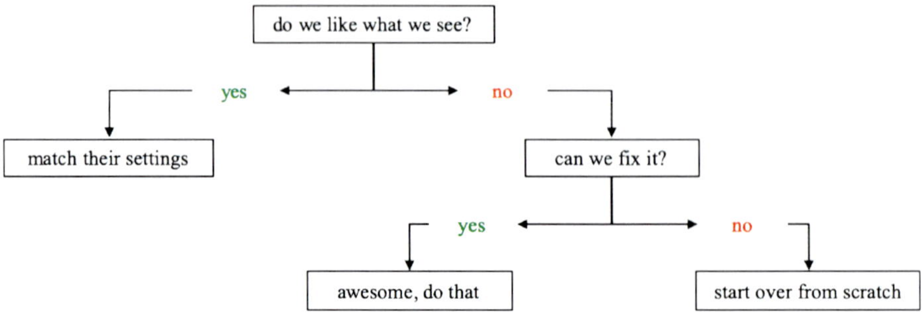

The first step in this little algorithm, "do we like what we see?" refers to a few different things: First of all are the **Three Big Things**: oxygenation, ventilation, and comfort – those for sure need to be addressed. Second is strategy: are the chosen settings at odds with what we had in mind? In the case of a hypovolemic patient with a high respiratory rate, for example, we may say, "yes, this strategy may be detrimental to the patient." In the case of an asthmatic patient with an I:E ratio of 1:3 we may decide, "this isn't what I would've set up from scratch, but let's see if it is working for the patient or not before deciding to change things." The idea here is to see what puts our patient at risk and what doesn't: a high percentage of time at decreased preload (%TaDP) and hypotension does put a patient at risk, while an I:E ratio of 1:3 in an asthmatic with no AutoPEEP doesn't.[259]

So we addressed the Three Big Things, we made sure the existing strategy isn't counterproductive based on what is going on with the patient, then we look at vitals and labs. The idea is to ensure that both perfusion and acid-base balance are all good, in the context of our vent strategy, and that we don't identify a life-threatening value or pattern of values with whatever information we have available. No need to get into specifics here, but if all is well in each of those general three subject areas, then there is no reason for us to go messing with settings and we should match what they are using.[260] The only exception here is if our machine can't do the settings they have. For example, if the patient is on **Pressure-Regulated Volume Control** and we don't have that choice, then we match their settings as best we can in either **Volume Control** or **Pressure Control** and go from there.

---

[259] To review these concepts: I:E ratio was in **Inspiratory Time (and I:E Ratio)**, percentage of time at decreased preload (%TaDP) was in **Hypotension**, and **AutoPEEP** in this context was in **Obstruction**

[260] And to brush up on blood gas interpretation, navigate to any of the following resources:
Woodruff, 2007 – Article that outlines a six-step approach to arterial blood gas interpretation
Smith, 2014 – Short video to review the basics of blood gas interpretation; while he uses kPa versus mmHg to outline normal values, it's the best of this type we've been able to find
Strong, 2014 – Much more detailed video series on the subject of arterial blood gasses

I:E – inspiratory to expiratory; **kPa** – kilopascal; **mmHg** – millimeters of mercury; **OK** – alright

But what about checking a **Plateau Pressure** and **AutoPEEP**? If our patient is alive and well and passes an assessment in all three categories we just discussed (the Three Big Things, vent strategy, vitals and labs), then those things can wait until we get them on to our vent. Some reasons for this: the delay here is only a few minutes at most, the measurements may vary by machine (i.e. how individual breaths are delivered), and we've already determined that the patient is stable via a number of different assessment parameters. And while scene time may or may not be a valid reason, we do want to use time efficiently and get patients moved unless we have reason to delay.

Let's redraw that algorithm we started with and add in just a little bit of detail to include all of these ideas. Then we'll move on to the next question and talk about it further:

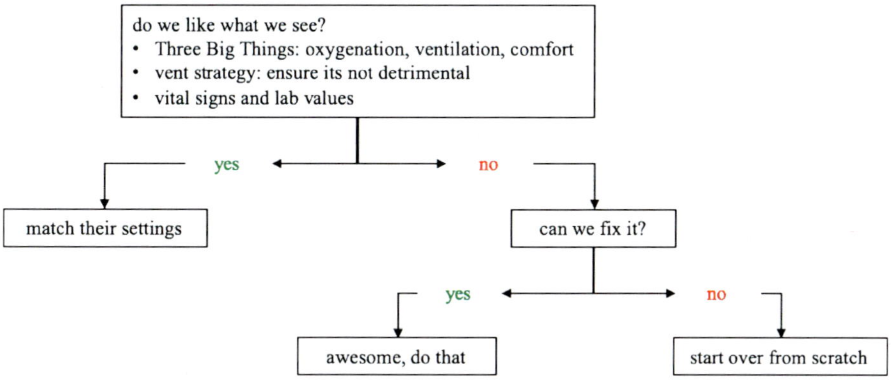

Next question to discuss further is, "can we fix it?" We'd like to address whatever issues we have (as determined by our assessment in the first box of the algorithm) by way of one or two interventions and keeping the majority of settings as they are.[261] For examples: if the patient is uncomfortable and we can provide analgesia on top of the sedation they are already getting, that may be all that is needed; if we can fix a high $EtCO_2$ by increasing **Tidal Volume** (or **Respiratory Rate**) a bit, no need to change mode or control; if we can address a potential for hypotension by decreasing rate and then increasing tidal volume, all is good; etc.[262] If, however, we are getting into a situation where it will take lots of changes to set things right, it may make the most sense to start from scratch with a whole new set of parameters. And in that case we may as well change a bunch of things and go with our preferences.

One thing worth mentioning here is that it is sometimes cool for us to make these changes as the patient lies and on the sending facility's (or crew's) machine. Other times we make adjustments as we transition to our machine. We for sure want to avoid alienating the transferring staff by messing with their machine if that relationship doesn't exist, so just be cognizant that are two sub-options in the "awesome, do that" course of action: do it right now and on their machine or do it as we transition on to our machine. Last thing and probably already obvious is that there is some middle ground here: we may make some changes right away and then defer other things until transfer, all as part of the same strategy. Example: give sedation now, adjust tidal volume or rate during the transition.

---

[261] And for help in deciding what vent changes to make, consider using Critical-Medical Guide – it's an app that's got a nifty feature in which we simply enter in current vent settings and an $EtCO_2$ goal and it spits out suggested vent changes

[262] We discussed these things in the sections on **Comfort**, **Ventilation**, and **Hypotension**

AutoPEEP – intrinsic positive end-expiratory pressure; **$EtCO_2$** – end-tidal carbon dioxide

And one more time, let's see how the algorithm would look with these additional details added in:

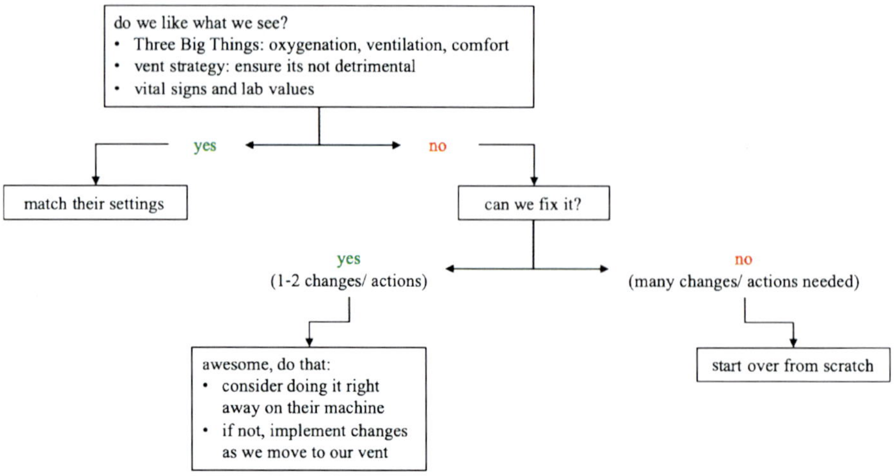

If at any time during this whole process things get too weird, we can always skip ahead to the "start over from scratch" end of things. Just recognize that the more changes we make, the less able we are to evaluate the efficacy of a single intervention. Like a science experiment, it helps to isolate variables and know that the observed result can be attributed to a specific adjustment. And even though we mentioned it already, interpersonal dynamics also come into play here: make changes based on necessity, not on personal preference. That will help maintain positive relationships with referring staff and crews.

I:E – inspiratory to expiratory; **kg** – kilograms; **ml** – milliliters; **PEEP** – positive end-expiratory pressure; **PIP** – peak inspiratory pressure; **Pplat** – plateau pressure

Keeping Things Going

This next section goes over what we do once we have the patient on our machine and the **Three Big Things** (oxygenation, ventilation, comfort) have all been addressed. We already talked about how we sometimes vary from the settings we start out at and this section explains how that happens. We want to both avoid injury and optimize air delivery, so we make adjustments to work towards those goals.

Watching Pressures

We discussed these things already, but here they are again: **Peak Inspiratory Pressure**, **Plateau Pressure**, **AutoPEEP**, **Mean Airway Pressure**, and **Driving Pressure**. And for visualization, in case we forgot, here's what they look like on a pressure waveform in **Volume Control** ventilation:

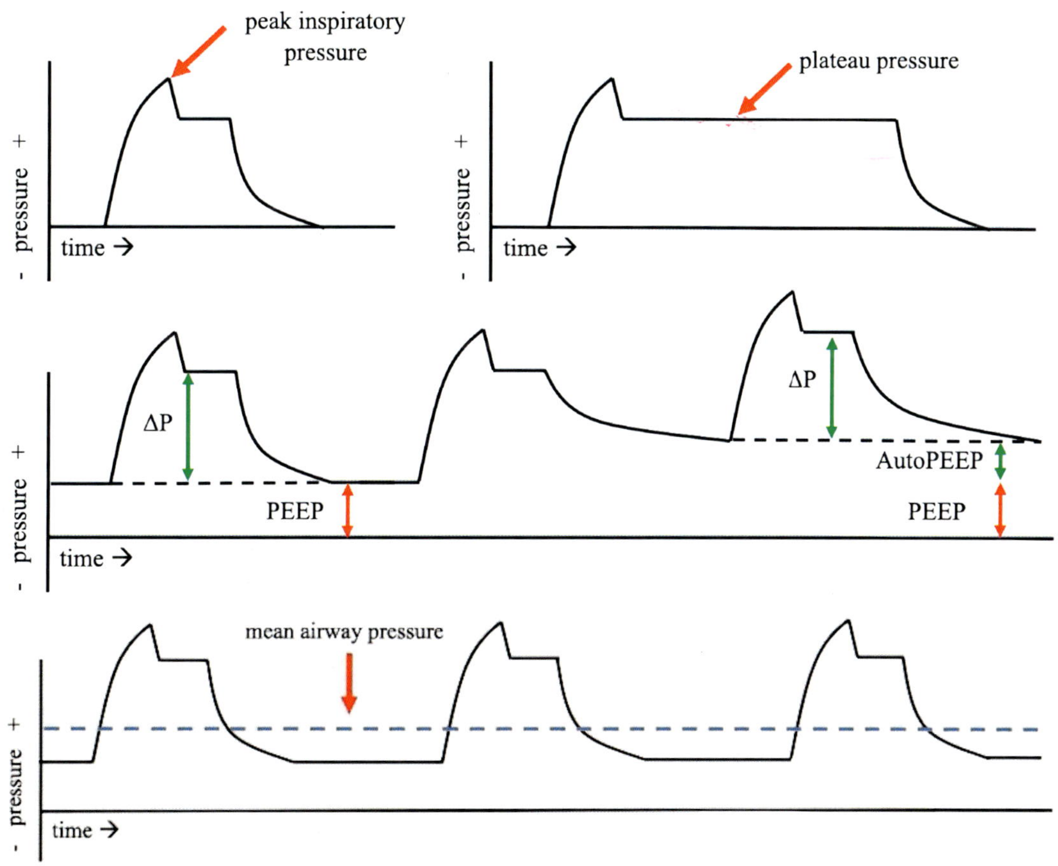

ΔP – driving pressure; **ARDS** – acute respiratory distress syndrome; **AutoPEEP** – intrinsic positive end-expiratory pressure; **cmH$_2$O** – centimeters of water

High for peak inspiratory pressure is 35cmH$_2$0, although we may go beyond that in certain situations (such as a small endotracheal tube). Plateau pressure max is normally 30cmH$_2$O and we do try to stick by that one whenever possible except in those cases where plateau pressure may not reflect alveolar pressure.[263] AutoPEEP is normally zero; we generally take actions to address AutoPEEP when we see evidence of it, but may tolerate a small amount before doing so. As for mean airway pressure, we don't generally cite a normal range, but know that a change in this value can be the first indicator of an alteration somewhere in the system. And driving pressure is most relevant with **Lung Injury**; in those cases we try to limit it to 15cmH$_2$O. All of these parameters should be checked (when possible, depending on control and patient's respiratory effort) within the first few minutes after placing someone on our machine and then again periodically through transport.[264] It may help to simply add these pressures on to a mental list of vital signs to reassess as we go.

As far as what to do with this information once we have it, here's a flowchart to help sift through the information and take action to address potential problems:[265]

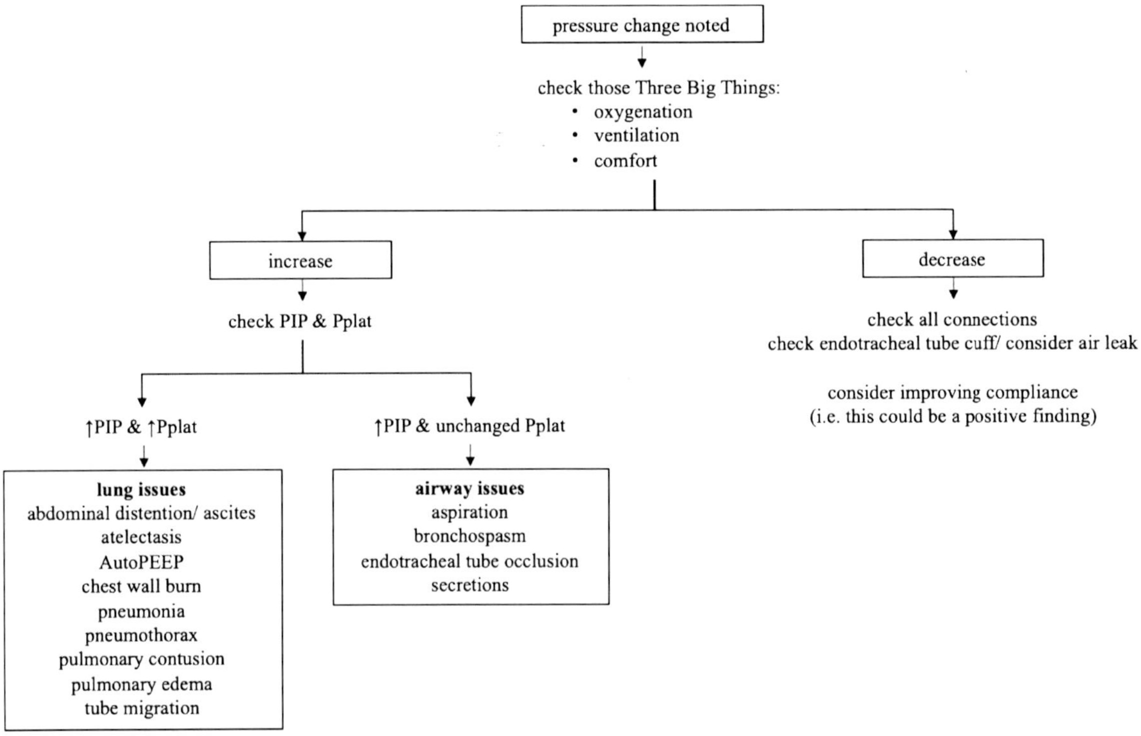

---

[263] We talked about these situations in **Plateau Pressure**, but just to reiterate: we assume plateau pressure is a reflection of alveolar pressure, but things that impede lung expansion can also give a high value

[264] For example, if a patient is triggering lots of breaths, we may not be able to get an AutoPEEP/ do an expiratory hold; if they are in pressure control ventilation, we may not be able to do an inspiratory hold (due to limitations of a particular machine)

[265] Lodeserto, 2018 – The left bit of this chart is similar to one he puts forth in his series on vent management

I:E – inspiratory to expiratory; **kg** – kilograms; **ml** – milliliters; **PEEP** – positive end-expiratory pressure; **PIP** – peak inspiratory pressure; **Pplat** – plateau pressure

And then let's look at potential solutions for each of these cases:[266] [267]

lung issues	
abdominal distention/ ascites	reposition or elevate head of bed
atelectasis	recruit some alveoli (via PEEP and/or recruitment maneuvers)
AutoPEEP	decrease I:E ratio, trial volume control, maybe adjust PEEP, disconnect circuit
chest wall burn	escharotomy
pneumonia	utilize PEEP to displace fluid
pneumothorax	remove from vent; needle decompression, chest tube, or finger thoracotomy
pulmonary contusion	consider lung injury strategy
pulmonary edema	utilize PEEP to displace fluid
tube migration	deflate cuff, pull back, re-inflate

airway issues	
aspiration	suction (prevent further aspiration), consider lung injury strategy
bronchospasm	fix with drugs, implement obstruction strategy
endotracheal tube occlusion	address comfort (biting), swap tube (something stuck)
secretions	suction

In **Pressure Control** ventilation when we may not have access to plateau pressure to identify these trends, there are other parameters we can look at. Most obvious is exhaled tidal volume: as compliance decreases, exhaled tidal volumes will drop (and vice versa).[268] In the case of airway obstruction, oftentimes we won't notice initially because the machine essentially accommodates for this increased airway resistance by using less flow:

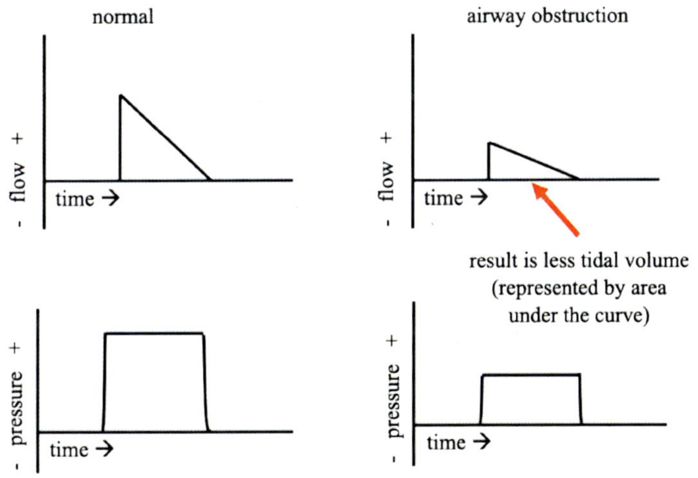

[266] Briggs & Freese, 2018 – There are also lots of weird cases out there to explain things that can happen, the chart above should not be assumed to be an exhaustive list of causes or fixes; as an example, this referenced article outlines a case of high airway pressures related to an endotracheal tube positioned with the bevel up against the wall of the trachea - the fix here was simply to rotate the tube 90 degrees

[267] And to link back to sections listed in this graphic: **Positive End-Expiratory Pressure**, **Inspiratory Time (and I:E Ratio)**, **Volume Control**, **Lung Injury**, **Comfort**, and **Obstruction**

[268] And to review this idea of monitoring compliance in pressure control ventilation, refer back to **Compliance (and Resistance)**

ΔP – driving pressure; **ARDS** – acute respiratory distress syndrome; **AutoPEEP** – intrinsic positive end-expiratory pressure; **cmH_2O** – centimeters of water

Since we don't typically monitor waveforms with transport ventilators, an airway obstruction may not get noticed in pressure control ventilation until it is severe enough to impact exhaled minute volume.[269] The best way to catch these sort of things before they have an impact on patient outcome is by setting alarms appropriately so that we are notified right away as things change (see following section).

Alarms[270] [271]

Next on our list of things to discuss are alarms. We won't talk about all the alarms that our machines might have, but we will talk about a few of the important ones. We can break alarms down into two general categories: ones that are default on the machine and ones that we set. Those default ones may be different between machines, but deliver similar messages like, "hey friend, our circuit got disconnected" and "oh snap, we ran out of oxygen." Those ones can be referenced and learned about in the manual for whatever machine we happen to be using. The other ones, the ones that we set, are the ones we'll focus on here.

One important alarm we set on the machine is the high-pressure alarm (which goes off when our high-pressure limit is reached). The reason this alarm is so important is that if it gets triggered, inspiration cycles off. That means that if we have a situation where we repeatedly trigger a high-pressure alarm, we may end up with a **Minute Volume** that bottoms out and a patient that quickly deteriorates. Imagine we place a patient on the vent who has either an untreated airway obstruction or poor compliance. If we try to ventilate this patient in **Volume Control** and at normal settings, every breath that goes in might trigger the high-pressure alarm and get terminated early with a net result of almost no minute volume. The reason this safeguard exists, in spite of this risk, is because we could for sure cause a lot of damage if we accidentally give too much pressure.

Moral of the story here: if we are in volume control ventilation and have a concern for increased airway pressures, we should consider going up on the high-pressure limit before putting the patient on the machine to avoid dropping our minute volume. On the flip side, in **Pressure Control** we need to vigilantly monitor exhaled minute volume (and also exhaled tidal volume) to avoid the same issue (of decreased minute volume). This leads us to the next most important alarm we can set: low minute volume. We set this limit at a reasonable value below our minute volume goal so that if things get weird and minute volume starts to drop, we get notified right away before our patient suffers. In this way, we utilize the high-pressure and low minute volume alarms to simultaneously ensure both safety and adequate ventilation for our patients.

---

[269] We can also (again, this is in pressure control) look at flow as calculated and delivered automatically by the vent; higher flows mean less resistance, so even if we don't know ranges or normal values we can still use this concept to trend changes

[270] Disclaimer about this section: there isn't much out there in the universe to provide guidance on how we should set these alarms; there are studies that have collected data on alarm settings for in-patient units, but we don't feel it would be appropriate to apply those to the transport setting; given that we move these patients one at a time with one or two providers (versus a unit full of vented patients, lots of alarms at once, and higher patient ratios) we should arguably always have eyes on the machine and it makes sense to use much tighter limits for alarms than we might see in the hospital setting; that said, this is just one opinion on the whole thing

[271] Weingart, 2019 – And for an alternative discussion of alarms which has some similarities to this one, refer to this podcast which advocates for treating all vent alarms as a "code blue" in the hospital setting

I:E – inspiratory to expiratory; **kg** – kilograms; **ml** – milliliters; **PEEP** – positive end-expiratory pressure; **PIP** – peak inspiratory pressure; **Pplat** – plateau pressure

As far as setting the high-pressure and low minute volume alarms, that is a bit dependent on our margin of safety and when we want to be notified of changes in the system. As a general rule of thumb, the high-pressure limit should be no more than $10cmH_2O$ above our **Peak Inspiratory Pressure**. If, however, our peak pressure is already high of normal, consider setting the high-pressure alarm $5cmH_2O$ over that value or at our upper limit of $35cmH_2O$:

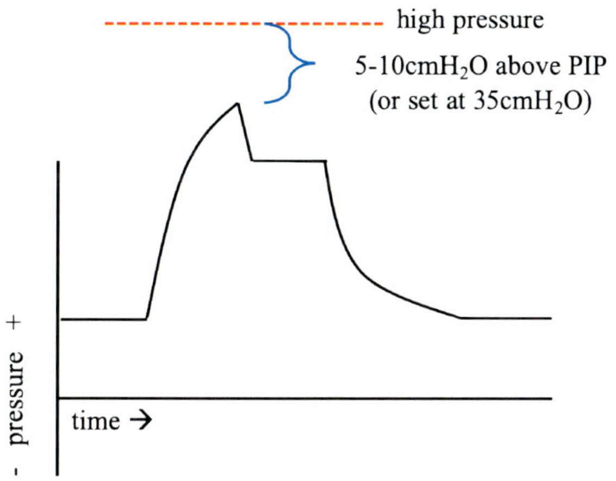

In the event of one of those situations which may lead to repeated triggering of the high-pressure alarm and sudden drop in minute volume, increase the high-pressure limit (even beyond $35cmH_2O$ if need be) to maintain minute volume. Note that this would be a short-term fix and we should start to consider other strategies right away: trial pressure control, consider pharmacologic and procedural interventions, etc.

As for the low minute volume alarm: set that within 25% of the minute volume goal that we calculated when we first started into this process of getting the patient on the vent.[272] If we have a patient breathing in excess of that goal and we want to know if that changes, we just set the low minute volume alarm 25% below what they are currently at. In any case, the low minute volume alarm is just a catch to alert us when we've missed a change. Typically we will be on top of these trends and notice things before the alarm even gets sounded, but sometimes we get distracted by other interventions and this backup system can keep us informed.

[272] And this 25% figure for where to set the low minute volume alarm is an arbitrary number that we feel is appropriate, there aren't too many specific recommendations for this type of thing

ΔP – driving pressure; **ARDS** – acute respiratory distress syndrome; **AutoPEEP** – intrinsic positive end-expiratory pressure; **cmH_2O** – centimeters of water

Other alarms that we can set to help us better keep track of what's going on with the vent and our patient are low peak-pressure, low frequency, high frequency, and low PEEP. Low peak-pressure alerts us when the peak inspiratory pressure is lower than we would expect; this could indicate a cuff leak, increase in patient's respiratory effort (i.e. negative pressure produced with patient effort), or a loose connection (an actual disconnection would probably trigger a disconnect alarm, one of those non-adjustable alarms consistent across machines, as the pressure would drop much more significantly). Low frequency can let us know if the patient's **Respiratory Rate** starts to decrease. This is good if the patient is consistently breathing above a set rate and we want to be aware if that intrinsic effort changes. And reasonably enough, the high-frequency alarm advises us when the patient starts to breathe faster or if some mishap is causing the machine to think that (s)he is. Lastly, low PEEP lets us know if the end-expiratory pressure drops below our set **Positive End-Expiratory Pressure**. This could indicate a leak, cuff deflation, or even an uncuffed tube (with pediatrics) that is too small.

That's just a quick overview of alarms; recognize that the most important ones are high pressure and low minute volume, but that there are a number that can help us be aware of changes in the system as we work through a transport. Because there is so much variation between machines, the best way to get familiar with the alarms we will be working with is to read the manual that comes with the machine. Super fun reading, but it's good information and can help us fine-tune the feedback from the vent so that we can better monitor what's going with the patient.

And we'll end with a graphic to show how some of these alarms would be represented on that pressure over time waveform in volume control ventilation:

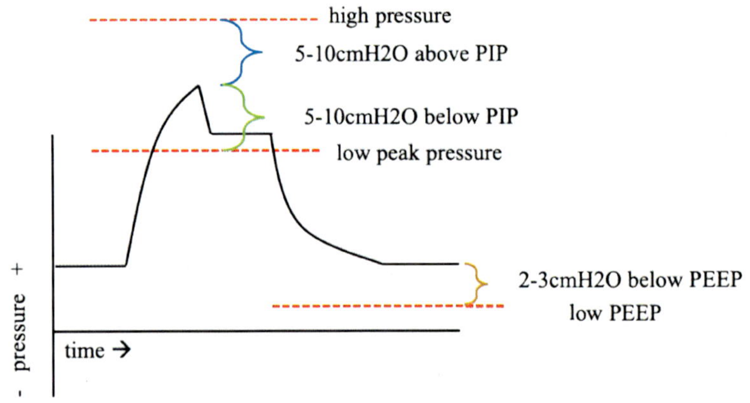

I:E – inspiratory to expiratory; **kg** – kilograms; **ml** – milliliters; **PEEP** – positive end-expiratory pressure; **PIP** – peak inspiratory pressure; **Pplat** – plateau pressure

Titrating Up on Tidal Volume?

Up to this point we've recommended considering **Tidal Volume** above that 6-8ml/kg range in just a few circumstances: to increase minute volume (in the **Ventilation** section), with airway **Obstruction**, and as part of the **Hypotension** strategy. But along the way we've mentioned that **Dead Space** is less than ideal and that more tidal volume is preferred to a higher respiratory rate. We also said that more breaths over an arbitrary amount of time means more of both that percentage of time at decreased preload (%TaDP) concept and stress on the system. Given all of these things, why would we not advocate for a higher tidal volume, lower respiratory rate strategy in all patients? The answer to that question isn't completely clear, but we'll try and answer it as best we can.

First thing to realize is that much of what we know about vent management these days is based on the ARDSNet study that compared a tidal volume of 6ml/kg to one of 12ml/kg with pretty significant findings.[273] Since then, most of the research out there has focused on this lung-protective approach. While there have been a few studies that looked at this middle ground of 8-10ml/kg, there's been no clear benefit over the 6ml/kg approach, so the default response is that we should stick with what we know works.[274] Which makes sense, but it doesn't consider the fact that there are multiple methods by which we can ensure safety while using more volume. For arguments sake, let's outline all of the things we can do mitigate the risks of a larger tidal volume and then we'll get back to this discussion.

First thing is that we want to limit our **Plateau Pressure** to a safe level below $30cmH_2O$ whenever possible, which includes when we decide to go up on tidal volume. Another concept we discussed was **Driving Pressure**. We mentioned in that section that most of the data on driving pressure is specific to the ARDS population, but also noted that there may be a case for using the value to guide treatment for patients in general. So let's just say that we want to limit driving pressure to $15cmH_2O$ as we outlined for the **Lung Injury** patients. Another component to consider, which we discussed in **Recruitment Maneuvers**, is that we prefer to make these types of changes in small increments and with as much time as possible between titrations. And lastly, we can utilize **Compliance** to help guide us towards our goal.

---

[273] The ARDS Network, 2000 – We cited this previously in the intro to **Specific Vent Strategies** and also in **Lung Injury**; this study is what led us all down the path of lung-protective ventilation in the first place

[274] Writing Group for the PReVENT Investigators, 2018 – This is one such study that attempted to investigate an intermediate tidal volume range; we previously cited a review of this article, but here it is as published

ΔP – driving pressure; **ARDS** – acute respiratory distress syndrome; **AutoPEEP** – intrinsic positive end-expiratory pressure; **cmH_2O** – centimeters of water

In **Volume Control** we could increase tidal volume until we notice a spike in **Plateau Pressure** or a decrease in compliance. In pressure control we increase pressure until we see a decrease in compliance or no increase in exhaled tidal volume after the adjustment. Once we hit either of these limits, we then titrate back the last increase (of tidal volume or pressure control) to where things were just before the previous adjustment. To map it all out with steps in the chart representing reassessment during transport:

volume control example				
step #	**tidal volume (ml)**	**plateau pressure (cmH_2O)**	**compliance (ml/cmH_2O)**	**action**
1	500	15	50	increase tidal volume
2	525	16	48	increase tidal volume
3	550	16	50	increase tidal volume
4	575	21	36	decrease tidal volume
5	550	16	50	no change, monitor
6	550	14	61	increase tidal volume

Note that even though plateau pressure doesn't get up to our previously established limit of $30cmH_2O$, we recognize that an increase beyond a tidal volume of 550 (line 4) gave us a spike in plateau pressure and drop in compliance. Therefore we may titrate back a smidge and wait for the lungs to fill more before moving back up (line 6).

And as for a how it looks in pressure control:

pressure control example				
step #	**pressure control (cmH_2O)**	**exhaled tidal volume (ml)**	**compliance (ml/cmH_2O)**	**action**
1	10	500	50	increase pressure control
2	11	550	50	increase pressure control
3	12	550	46	increase pressure control (or stay)
4	13	550	42	decrease pressure control
5	12	550	46	no change, monitor
6	12	600	50	increase pressure control

Exhaled tidal volume and compliance will likely vary from breath to breath and therefore it isn't quite as easy to recognize these trends in real-time, but the general idea holds true.

To get back to our original argument about titrating up on tidal volume: recognizing the fact that going up on tidal volume would allow us to go down on respiratory rate with the result of less dead space and less stress into the system, it intuitively makes sense to consider how we can go about making this happen in a manner that is as safe as possible. Firstly we will want to limit plateau pressure to less than $30cmH_2O$. Next we may want to limit driving pressure to $15cmH_2O$ even though that recommendation is normally reserved for ARDS patients. Beyond that we can make changes to tidal volume in small and incremental steps while simultaneously monitoring changes to plateau pressure and/ or compliance with each adjustment.

I:E – inspiratory to expiratory; **kg** – kilograms; **ml** – milliliters; **PEEP** – positive end-expiratory pressure; **PIP** – peak inspiratory pressure; **Pplat** – plateau pressure

Given that all of these precautions to ensure safety are in place, we propose that going up on tidal volume is probably just fine for our vented patients once all the other issues have been worked through. That said, there are a few more things to mention. First is that this process takes time and many transports will exclude this level of detail in ventilator management. Second is that upper limits to plateau pressure and driving pressure are not rigid guidelines, rather they indicate endpoints at which risk clearly outweighs benefit. To say it another way, just because a plateau pressure is 28 or a driving pressure is 13, both below established upper limits, doesn't mean it that is as comparably safe as having a plateau pressure of 23 or a driving pressure of 11. And last thing to mention: there is no evidence that going up on tidal volume in this manner would change patient outcome in any direction, it's just something to think about and consider at this point.

ABC – airway, breathing, circulation; **ARDS** – acute respiratory distress syndrome;
AutoPEEP – intrinsic positive end-expiratory pressure; **BLS** – basic life support; **BVM** – bag valve mask;
CPR – cardiopulmonary resuscitation; **DOPE** – displaced tube, obstruction, pneumothorax, equipment;
DOTTS – disconnect the vent circuit, ~~O_2 100% via BVM~~, tube position or function, tweak vent, sonography

Acute Deterioration

The next thing to chat about is what to do if the patient begins to decompensate while on the vent. Let's start with a common memory tool to address some of the major causes of acute deterioration of the mechanically ventilated patient:

the DOPE mnemonic		
	issue	**action**
D	displaced tube	confirm tube placement
O	obstruction	suction, check for kinked endotracheal tube, consider bronchospasm
P	pneumothorax	remove patient from vent; decompress, chest tube, or finger thoracotomy
E	equipment	check all connections

There are also some variations of this guy, so we may see it out there with an "S" at the end for stacking (i.e. **AutoPEEP**),[275] an "R" at the end for rigidity of the chest wall (a rare complication of Fentanyl administration),[276] or even with the "P" to represent pain and/ or (Auto)PEEP.[277] It is also sometimes accompanied by another mnemonic called DOTTS which outlines actions that can be taken to fix issues identified by DOPE. Now DOTTS includes a step where we bag the patient with a bag-valve mask (BVM) and we've crossed that step out. We don't recommend routinely taking someone off the vent unless we have good reason to and we'll get back to this idea in just a little bit. But just so we can see it in its true representation, here it is:[278]

the DOTTS mnemonic		
	action	**explanation**
D	disconnect the vent circuit	to fix AutoPEEP or decreased preload (i.e. pneumothorax or hypotension)
~~**O**~~	~~O_2 100% via BVM~~	~~to manually assess for issues (i.e. look, listen, feel)~~
T	tube position or function	includes assessing placement and suctioning
T	tweak vent	consider decreasing rate, tidal volume, or inspiratory time (i.e. with AutoPEEP or hypotension)
S	sonography	consider ultrasound to identify issues (if we have it)

[275] Rezaie, 2018 – Describes the "S" added to the DOPE mnemonic; also gives on overview of the DOTTS idea discussed below
[276] Thomas & Abraham, 2018 – While the "R" component to the DOPE mnemonic isn't all that common, it may be worth keeping in mind
[277] Wright, 2014 – A great read on ARDS in general, but specific to this cause he's got a nice DOPE graphic that he adapted from another source
[278] To link back to sections mentioned in this chart: **Hypotension**, **Respiratory Rate**, **Tidal Volume**, and **Inspiratory Time (and I:E Ratio)**

EMS – emergency medical services; **$EtCO_2$** – end-tidal carbon dioxide; **FiO_2** – fraction of inspired oxygen **I:E** – inspiratory to expiratory; **MV** – minute volume; **O_2** – oxygen; **PaO_2** – partial pressure of arterial oxygen; **PEEP** – positive end-expiratory pressure; **PIP** – peak inspiratory pressure; **Pplat** – plateau pressure; **SpO_2** pulse oximetry

The DOPE mnemonic (with or without DOTTS) is easy to remember and can be used to guide the initial troubleshooting process when the patient starts to deteriorate.[279] Many of these occurrences can be tied to **Alarms** or other assessment parameters, but that depends on which type of machine we are working on and what tools we have available. For example, a tube displaced too deep will give a high-pressure alarm (and eventually a low minute volume alarm) and a tube displaced out of the airway will likely result in a low-pressure alarm. In regard to other assessments: a tube displaced too deep will lead to a high **Mean Airway Pressure** or **Peak Inspiratory Pressure**, low exhaled tidal volume, patient discomfort, etc. and a tube displaced out of the airway causes a low mean airway pressure, drop in $EtCO_2$ with change in waveform, hypoxia, etc.

Because there are so many things to consider, building an algorithm to troubleshoot each possibility gets a bit difficult. We'll go ahead and do it anyway, we just need to consider a few more things in preparation. First of all is that acute deterioration of the vented patient doesn't always mean that there is an issue with the vent, it could be some other issue beyond the vent (i.e. endotracheal tube displaced or pathophysiologic process). If it's a vent thing, then we mess around with the vent; but if it's another issue, our interventions should focus on drugs and procedures and that sort of thing. Think of it this way:

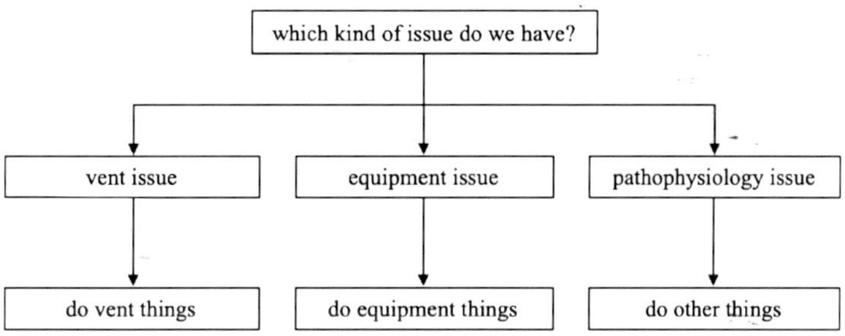

Now the reality is that it isn't always so cut and dry. There are times where we do both vents things and other things simultaneously. An example of this would be a patient already on the vent who experiences an allergic reaction to something. In this case we could simultaneously proceed with an **Obstruction** vent strategy and give drugs to fix the problem. So while our little algorithm may be too simple, it often helps to take a moment to think about which sort of problem we have on hand and act accordingly.

---

[279] Weingart, 2011 – For some trivia on where the DOPE mnemonic came from, take a look here

ABC – airway, breathing, circulation; **ARDS** – acute respiratory distress syndrome;
AutoPEEP – intrinsic positive end-expiratory pressure; **BLS** – basic life support; **BVM** – bag valve mask;
CPR – cardiopulmonary resuscitation; **DOPE** – displaced tube, obstruction, pneumothorax, equipment;
DOTTS – disconnect the vent circuit, ~~O_2 100% via BVM~~, tube position or function, tweak vent, sonography

In light of the fact that there are so many variables involved, here's the stepwise approach we suggest for troubleshooting acute deterioration of a ventilated patient. This approach takes advantage of feedback that we may have available to us from vent alarms and assessment parameters:[280]

acute deterioration: what to do!?

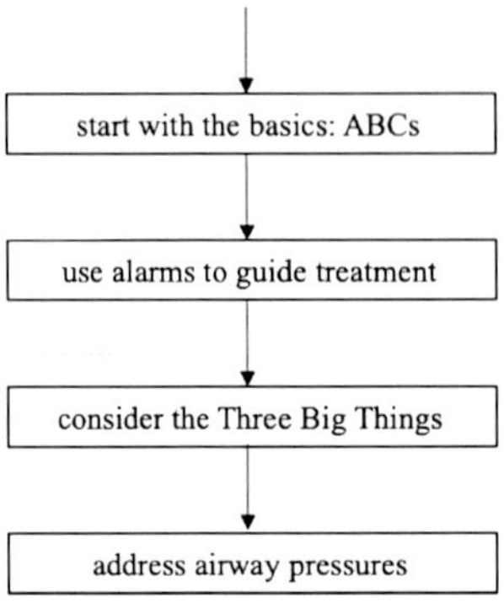

And in fact, one could argue that "use alarms to guide treatment" may even be a quicker solve than starting with the ABCs. While we recognize that this is blasphemy in the world of EMS and transport medicine, here's how that might look:

acute deterioration: what to do!?

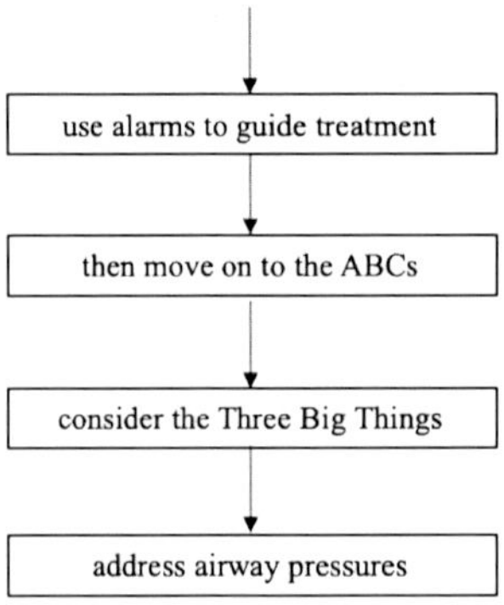

[280] And to refer back to these things: **Three Big Things**, **Keeping Things Going** (and specifically, **Alarms**)

EMS – emergency medical services; **EtCO$_2$** – end-tidal carbon dioxide; **FiO$_2$** – fraction of inspired oxygen
I:E – inspiratory to expiratory; **MV** – minute volume; **O$_2$** – oxygen; **PaO$_2$** – partial pressure of arterial oxygen;
PEEP – positive end-expiratory pressure; **PIP** – peak inspiratory pressure; **Pplat** – plateau pressure; **SpO$_2$** pulse oximetry

By working through each of these steps systematically, we hit all of the DOPE things and identify where in the system the issue lies (vent, equipment, physiology). Now, it gets a bit more complicated when we add in specifics for each step along the way, but remember that the basic idea is a simple set of four steps:[281]

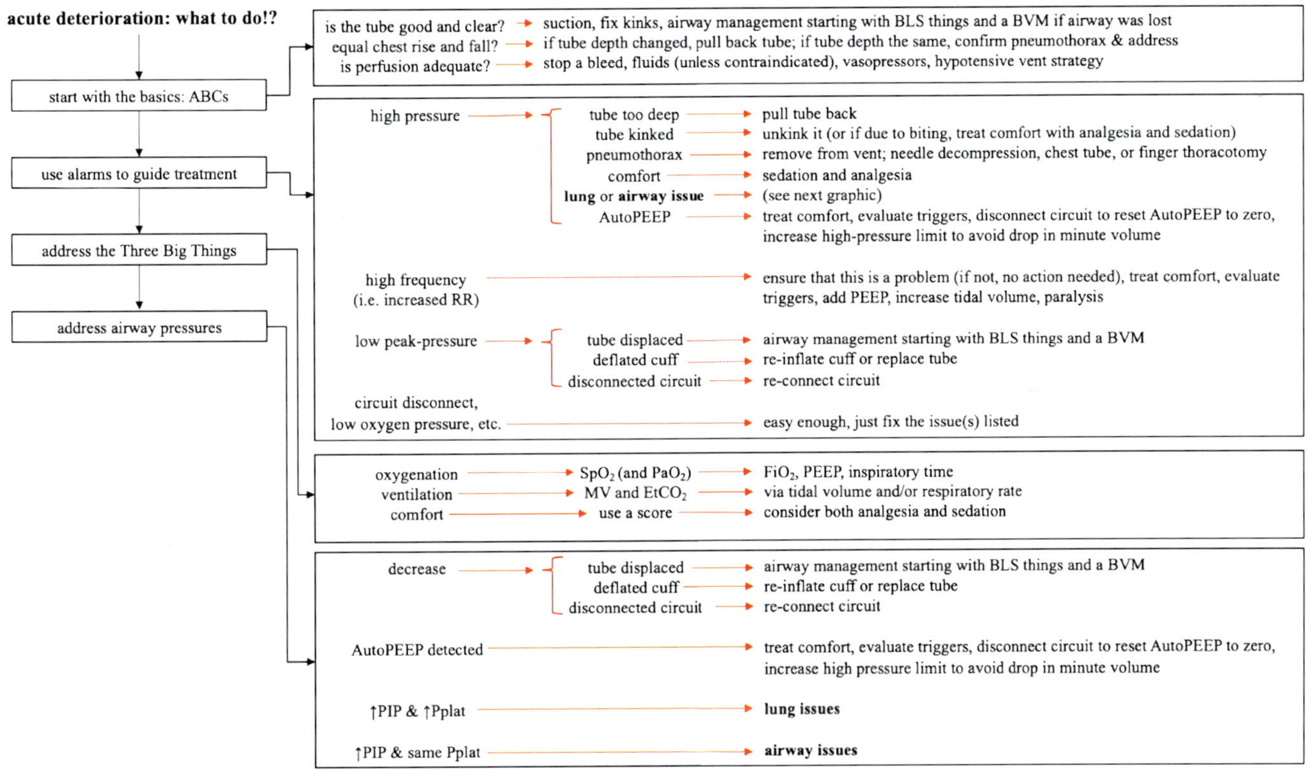

A few things to note about this algorithm: with a partially deflated cuff, remove air from the cuff and then re-inflate with an appropriate amount of air. Simply adding volume can contribute to both injury from over-inflation and likelihood of tube displacement.[282] Also consider using a monometer to measure cuff pressure and establish a baseline moving forward if available. And if the cuff is defective, consider utilizing a bougie to exchange it for a new one or take steps to fix the issue temporarily.[283]

---

[281] And refer back to **Vent Parameters, Round Two** to review the pressures
[282] Tennyson & friends, 2016 – This paper reviews the incidence of endotracheal tube cuff over-inflation in the helicopter EMS setting
[283] Mellick, 2014; Lauria & friends, 2019 – The first is a video that demonstrates exchanging a tube using a bougie; the second is a short article that outlines strategies for salvaging a damaged endotracheal tube

ABC – airway, breathing, circulation; **ARDS** – acute respiratory distress syndrome; **AutoPEEP** – intrinsic positive end-expiratory pressure; **BLS** – basic life support; **BVM** – bag valve mask; **CPR** – cardiopulmonary resuscitation; **DOPE** – displaced tube, obstruction, pneumothorax, equipment; **DOTTS** – disconnect the vent circuit, ~~O_2 100% via BVM~~, tube position or function, tweak vent, sonography

There's no way to accommodate all possibilities in a single algorithm without getting too crazy on the details, but that's the basic idea. Before moving on, just a few things to note. First is that a low minute volume alarm may also accompany acute deterioration, but it will likely be tied to either a high-pressure alarm (with breaths cycling off due to that alarm getting triggered) or some kind of disconnect (which would likely be indicated by a circuit disconnect or low peak-pressure alarm). We also didn't include a low-frequency or low-PEEP alarm anywhere in this flowchart, as those probably aren't tied to an acute deterioration unless accompanied by one of these other trump cards. And then we already showed this before (and recognize that not all of these are acute life threats), but just to clarify again the different lung and airway issues we might come across:

lung issues	
abdominal distention/ ascites	reposition or elevate head of bed
atelectasis	recruit some alveoli (via PEEP and/or recruitment maneuvers)
AutoPEEP	decrease I:E ratio, trial volume control, maybe adjust PEEP, disconnect circuit
chest wall burn	escharotomy
pneumonia	utilize PEEP to displace fluid
pneumothorax	remove from vent; needle decompression, chest tube, or finger thoracotomy
pulmonary contusion	consider lung injury strategy
pulmonary edema	utilize PEEP to displace fluid
tube migration	deflate cuff, pull back, re-inflate

airway issues	
aspiration	suction (prevent further aspiration), consider lung injury strategy
bronchospasm	fix with drugs, implement obstruction strategy
endotracheal tube occlusion	address comfort (biting), swap tube (something stuck)
secretions	suction

Now let's summarize what actions to take in the event of an acutely deteriorating patient on the vent. While there is a well-known memory tool (the DOPE mnemonic) to guide us through troubleshooting potential issues, that tool doesn't consider feedback from the machine (i.e. alarms) and, therefore, we suggest a simple sequence of four steps to work through it all: check the ABCs, look at and address any alarms, review the **Three Big Things**, then check pressures. If by then we haven't figured out our problem, we can consider taking the patient off the vent and bagging by hand (still not a great strategy though…) or getting out the ultrasound machine to try and identify an issue (if available).[284]

---

[284] Mojoli, 2017 – And for those of us who do have ultrasound, here's a short article that discusses application in mechanical ventilation

EMS – emergency medical services; **$EtCO_2$** – end-tidal carbon dioxide; **FiO_2** – fraction of inspired oxygen
I:E – inspiratory to expiratory; **MV** – minute volume; **O_2** – oxygen; **PaO_2** – partial pressure of arterial oxygen;
PEEP – positive end-expiratory pressure; **PIP** – peak inspiratory pressure; **Pplat** – plateau pressure; **SpO_2** pulse oximetry

The final idea here is what to do if the patient goes into cardiac arrest while on the vent. Standard practice in this situation is to take the patient off the vent and have someone ventilate by hand while CPR is initiated. That may be a valid option if we have extra hands, but in transport with only two clinicians it may not be possible. If our particular machine allows us to ventilate without patient triggers (i.e. in controlled mechanical ventilation or intermittent mandatory ventilation), that would be the preferred approach. If not, then we may be able to approximate those **Basic Modes of Ventilation** by maxing out the sensitivity of our trigger. The reason we turn off the mechanism for patient-triggered breaths is that the machine will likely be triggered to deliver a breath with each chest compression given.

Another consideration in this cardiac arrest situation is that we may need to increase our high-pressure limit so that breaths don't get cut short early during this time. If the machine is trying to give a breath while we are trying to simultaneously give compressions, we will most definitely exceed a normally-set high-pressure limit with the result that breaths will get cycled off. Ideally we could time our compressions with the machine's breaths to avoid this, but that would be difficult to accomplish. Increasing the high-pressure limit does predispose the patient to both barotrauma and increased intrathoracic pressure, but it may be the best course of action when working a code with limited resources.

One last recap and then we'll move on. With a deteriorating patient on the vent, try to keep it simple and work through four steps: ABCs, alarms, Three Big Things, and pressures. If after that you can't figure out the issue, consider removing the patient from the vent and bagging by hand (with a PEEP valve, if available). And if other assessment techniques such as ultrasound are available, they can also be used to further investigate causes of deterioration. In the event that the patient arrests while on the vent, cancel out patient-triggers and increase your high-pressure limit.

ARDS – acute respiratory distress syndrome; EKG – electrocardiogram

Additional Concepts, Round Two

Filters[285]

Filters are used in mechanical ventilation to prevent infectious gunk from transferring from one spot to another. In the transport setting we generally use in-line filters that simply fit into the vent circuit. While there are a few possible options as to where we place the filter, it is commonly put at the connection between the machine and the vent circuit (i.e. the inhalation side of the system):

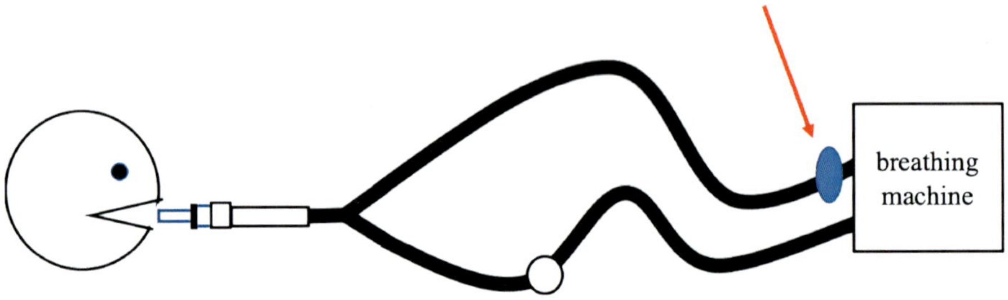

The filter placed here essentially keeps stuff at the machine from getting to the patient. Which is fine, just recognize that it doesn't keep bad stuff at the patient from getting to us and our coworkers:

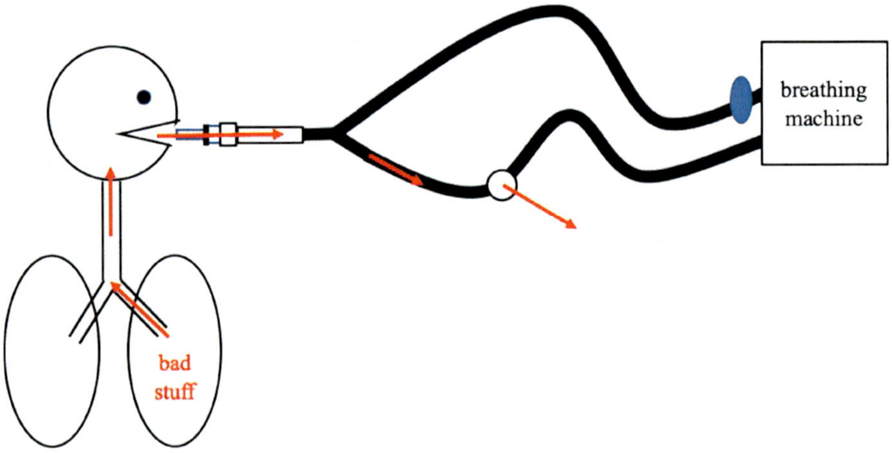

Now we could work around that by placing the filter at the patient's face/ endotracheal tube or even on the exhalation side of things, but the face option will increase mechanical dead space and the exhalation side option may not be available with our transport vent.[286] That said, placing a filter near the tube may be warranted in certain cases (tuberculosis, flu, etc.), just know that in addition to the dead space issue it can also impede the movement of air. But if we have a patient with something that we don't want to breathe in and neither of these strategies is appropriate or possible, be sure to mask up!

---

[285] Wilkes, 2011a & 2011b – He gives the most in-depth discussion of both filters (this section) and humidifiers (next section)

[286] The impact of adding the humidifier (and other devices) to the circuit is discussed in both **Dead Space** and the **Appendix**

HME – heat & moisture exchanger; **ml** – milliliter; **OK** – alright

Humidifiers[287 288]

Humidification of air is important in mechanical ventilation because dry air can cause damage to the lining of the respiratory tract. No need to get into the details here, just know that absent any contraindications we ought to try and add some degree of humidification to the air we push into the patient's lungs. We typically do this in transport by placing a humidification device called a heat & moister exchanger (HME) between the endotracheal tube and wye of the vent circuit. Placing the device further up on the inhalation side of the circuit would not work, as the device functions by trapping moisture (and also heat) from exhaled air and allowing it to be blown back into the patient's airways on the subsequent breath:

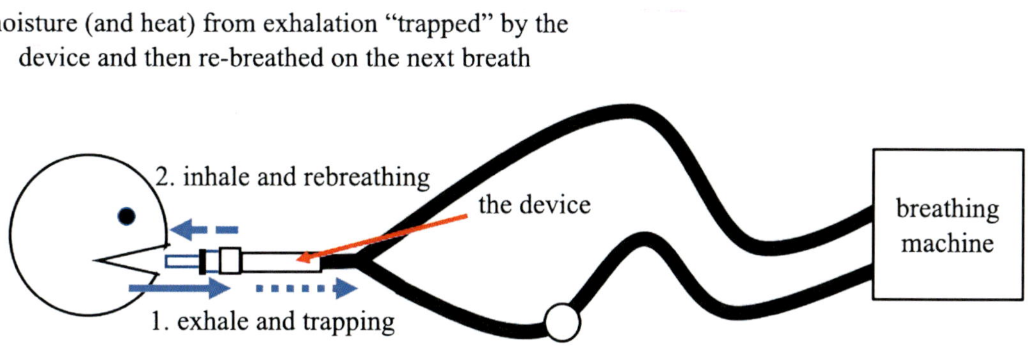

---

[287] Yartsev, 2019 – Navigate here for a discussion of the passive style devices used in the transport setting
[288] Gillies & friends, 2017 – This Cochrane Review has determined that passive humidifiers are comparable to actual humidification in providing therapeutic benefit and avoiding primary complications (airway obstruction, pneumonia, mortality); while they admit that more research is needed, it's good to know that these devices do have demonstrated value

ARDS – acute respiratory distress syndrome; **EKG** – electrocardiogram

The humidifier is often the biggest contributor to mechanical dead space (as outlined in the **Appendix**), but it ought to be used unless we have good reason not to. One of these good reasons not to would be a small **Tidal Volume**, such as with kids or **Lung Injury** patients.[289] In these situations, we want to minimize mechanical dead space as much as possible. Now there are smaller devices designed for pediatrics and here's the basic idea on that: humidifiers are rated to provide humidification for a certain amount of tidal volume; higher value corresponds with more space needed within the internals of the device and, therefore, more dead space.[290] To make this clear, let's look at info from one particular product line:[291]

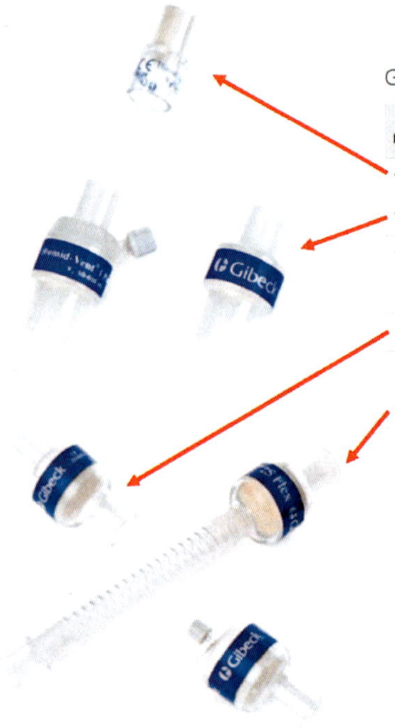

Gibeck® Humid-Vent® HME

ITEM CODE	DESCRIPTION	TV RANGE (ML)	MOISTURE OUTPUT (MG H2O/L)	WEIGHT (G)	RESISTANCE (CM H2O)	DEAD SPACE (ML)	CASE QUANTITY
10011	Humid-Vent Mini	15-50	30, Vt = 20 mL	4.5	0.9, 10 lpm	2.4	30
11112	Humid-Vent 1	50-600	30.5, Vt = 0.2 L	9.4	0.3, 20 lpm	10	50
11132	Humid-Vent 1 port	50-600	30.5, Vt = 0.2 L	11.6	0.3, 20 lpm	14	25
13312	Humid-Vent 2 port	150-1500	28, Vt = 0.6 L	20.9	0.8, 60 lpm	29	20
14412	Humid-Vent 2S	150-1500	28, Vt = 0.6 L	19.8	0.8, 60 lpm	29	20
17731	Humid-Vent 2S Flex–sterile	250-1500	28, Vt = 0.6 L	26.4	0.8, 60 lpm	54	20
17732	Humid-Vent 2S Flex–clean	250-1500	28, Vt = 0.6 L	26.4	0.8, 60 lpm	54	20

we see here that more capacity for humidification means more dead space

[289] Hinkson & friends, 2006 – This article looks at the effect of dead space in mechanically ventilated patients, we'll visit it again in the **Appendix** and will focus in on applying the idea to treatment of pediatric patients

[290] Which means we could theoretically use a smaller-sized humidifier for an adult patient ventilated via a low-volume strategy

[291] Teleflex, 2019 (images) – Just to be clear, no relationship or conflict of interest here; it's just really nice how they lay out all the product info like this for us to talk about

HME – heat & moisture exchanger; **ml** – milliliter; **OK** – alright

Second good reason not to use a humidifier would be the concurrent use of nebulized medications.[292] We want those drugs going into the patient, not getting absorbed by the device. While we could theoretically place the in-line nebulizer between the endotracheal tube and the humidifier, that would result in decreased medication administration unless we also added in a spacer. But then we'd have a huge amount of dead space and we already established that we want to cut down on that whenever possible. Also, the need for a humidifier is less with a nebulized medication because we are actively pushing moisture into the airways along with whatever medication is being given. It is, however, OK to remove the humidifier for administration of a nebulized drug and then reattach it as soon as that is done.

One other situation in which we ought to exercise concern with a humidifier would be increased secretions, as the device can get clogged up to the point where it impedes airflow. This isn't a case in which we never use a humidifier, rather it's one of those cases where we need to be aware of potential problems. Increases in **Peak Inspiratory Pressure** in **Volume Control** or decreases in exhaled tidal volume in **Pressure Control** would likely be our first indication of an airflow problem of this sort.[293] If this happens and we are worried about a humidifier getting clogged up, we can either remove the device or replace it with a fresh one.

Very last thing about humidifiers before moving on: while all of these devices provide some filtration of exhaled air, certain devices may even be classified as both a filter and a humidifier. This could potentially mitigate the escape of infectious material from the patient into the ambient air via the exhalation side of the vent circuit as we drew out in the last section.

---

[292] And see the very next section for a discussion of **In-line Nebulization**

[293] Since we don't routinely monitor flow in the transport setting, we instead have to look at other parameters to diagnose these kinds of air movement problems

ARDS – acute respiratory distress syndrome; **EKG** – electrocardiogram

In-line Nebulization

Just to demonstrate a few things about why we do nebs the way we do, let's look at a setup of how the system looks when we nebulize a medication through the vent circuit. Recognize that there may be some variation between models, this is just the setup with which we are most familiar with and serves to outline the important stuff:[294]

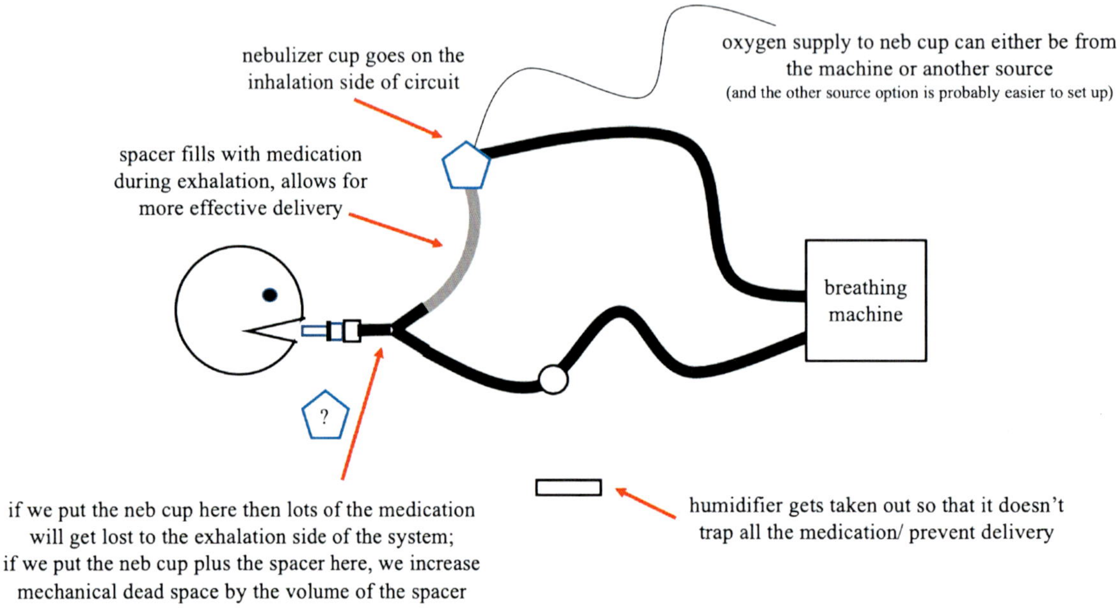

That should be clear enough, but just to expand on a few points: we may need adapters and extra vent tubing to make this work, so we should plan ahead and have that stuff available in pre-built kits. The spacer is important, as medication will be lost to the exhalation side of the circuit if it isn't there. Some machines recommend specific changes to settings to facilitate this process, read up on that or have a chat with the manufacturer's rep for details about a particular machine.

[294] Dhand, 2017 – And for more info on placement of the nebulizer and bias flow (which we don't get into here), take a read of this article

HME – heat & moisture exchanger; **ml** – milliliter; **OK** – alright

Prone Ventilation

Prone ventilation is when we lay our ventilated patient face down on the bed or stretcher. Arguments and evidence in favor of prone ventilation include things like better ventilation/ perfusion (V/Q) match, improved **Oxygenation**, more effective **Ventilation**, etc.[295] That said, prone ventilation isn't for everyone, studies are shrouded a bit by bias, and efficacy seems to be related to early implementation, time of application each day (16 hours per day!), and severity of hypoxemia (i.e. proning has benefit when oxygenation is a major issue).[296] When we are called to transport a pronated patient, there are some logistical limitations to the process. Much of what we do requires access to the patient's front side and many of the tools we use in medicine are designed with the supine patient in mind. All that said, it is likely that we will see more of this in years to come so it makes sense to do a quick survey as to where things are at in regard to prone ventilation in the field.

Prone ventilation has been mostly studied in patients with ARDS. Given that ARDS isn't something we commonly diagnose or come across initially on scene runs, it seems likely that most of our prone ventilation will be done in the context of interfacility transfers. Which is good, because the process of getting someone pronated with an endotracheal tube and vent in place isn't the fastest thing we could do and managing an airway on an already pronated presents its own complications. So interfacility transfers of ARDS folks seems to be where we will most likely be using this technique as critical care transport providers.

We mentioned before in our section on **Lung Injury** that recruitment of alveoli and maintenance of this recruitment is very important. While it may be tempting to simply flip a pronated patient over for transport and then let the receiving facility re-pronate them, this could potentially set progress back quite a bit, so we want to do what we can to keep our actions in line with overall clinical course. That said, many treatment guidelines or algorithms for this sort of thing include cyclical proning on some sort of schedule. It may be worth timing these transfers in line with transport capabilities (i.e. with no capacity to transport a prone patient, simply wait until it's supine time and make it happen then).[297]

---

[295] Koulouras & friends, 2016; Henderson & friends, 2014 – For details on the benefits of prone ventilation, take a look at either of these articles

[296] Bloomfield & friends, 2015 – Refer here for insight on research that has been done to date and recommendations for what ought to be investigated moving forward

[297] Olveira & friends, 2017 – And as one example of that, take a look at this protocol for prone ventilation; it also goes into detail on how to carry out the physical maneuver and discusses many of the concerns that could potentially arise along the way

ARDS – acute respiratory distress syndrome; **EKG** – electrocardiogram

When it comes to the physical process of flipping someone over, there are a number of techniques and tools than run the gamut from a RotoProne bed[298] to simply using a flat sheet or slider.[299] Proning can also be performed at the time of transfer from one bed or stretcher to another. For example, let's say we are going from a hospital that doesn't do this to one that does; we could facilitate this at either end of the transfer.[300] This means that even if we don't transport a patient in a prone position in our vehicle, we may still get caught up in the process at some point.

A few considerations about transporting a pronated patient: access to the airway may be difficult or impossible, access to the anterior chest wall (for EKGs, assessment of heart and lung sounds, needle thoracostomy, etc.) will be limited, and stretcher or sled configuration may dictate that the patient be horizontal. For all of these reasons (and probably a great many others), it may be quite some time until certain programs and crews decide to attempt this, but rest assured that it has been done already and will likely become more common in years to come.[301]

---

[298] Arjo, 2020 – Manufacturer's content on the RotoProne bed, just for those who are curious about it

[299] Critical Care & Major Trauma Network, 2015; Critical Care Cardiff, 2017 – Two YouTube videos that demonstrate proning a patient

[300] Hospital Direct, 2017 – Another YouTube video that shows the maneuver while moving a patient between surfaces

[301] Boon & Boon, 2018 – These guys have both transported prone patients and provide a good overview of its application in the transport setting; they also have a video at that same link that shows a one-person technique for flipping a patient on a stretcher

and since this section is a cheat-sheet of sorts that has almost all of the abbreviations,
we'll skip the legend here and direct readers back to the rest of the text

A Proposed Protocol/ Flowchart

The goal of this learning experience is that we will know enough about vents so that we can understand why we make changes and how those changes affect our patients. Working towards that end, it may help to have a framework to work with while managing a patient.[302] We've tried to create an algorithm that covers all we've talked about up to now, that is generic enough to apply to different machines, and that fits on two opposing pages so that it can easily be utilized as a reference in the field.[303] It's here to help folks work towards a higher level of competency or to simply take some of the load off of one's mind when things get busy on scene or in transport.

The basic idea of the flow is something like this:

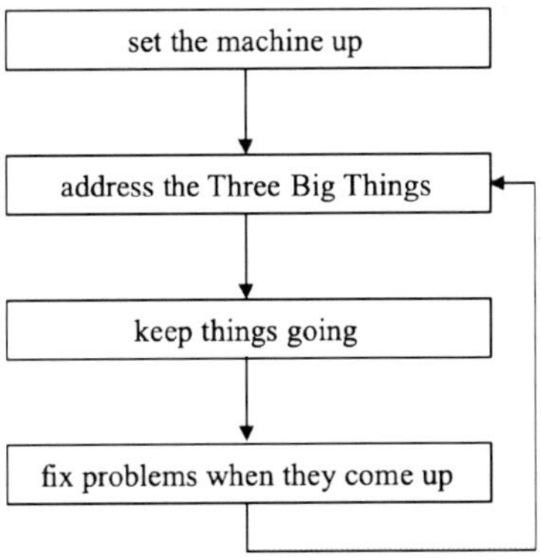

[302] Wright, 2014; Nagler & Chiefetz, 2019 – Throughout this manual we've cited a number of different resources, but here are two of them that summarize the steps of mechanical ventilation from start to finish; they vary somewhat from what we've outlined, but provide another perspective on moving through all the steps in a systematic fashion

[303] Weingart, 2010 – As another example, this document that accompanies the podcast series can also be used as a step by step guide in a similar way to one we've outlined here

How to do Vent Stuff

I. Set the Machine Up

IBW_{male} (kg) = (2.3(height in inches) – 60) + 50
IBW_{female} (kg) = (2.3(height in inches) – 60) + 45.5
TV = 6-8ml/kg
MV = 100ml/kg IBW/min

1. prep
   a. get a report from sending
   b. do some arithmetic: IBW, tidal volume, minute volume
   c. assess the patient
   d. consider a strategy
   e. check circuit, attach $EtCO_2$ and filter; consider need for humidifier and/ or suction

2. determine settings
   a. patient already on vent (see algorithm, right)
   b. from scratch
      i. turn on machine and leave at default mode and control
      ii. dial in desired tidal volume for 6ml/kg (or pressure control at 10-15cmH2O)
      iii. adjust respiratory rate
         1. adults: to minute volume goal
         2. kids: using a reference range
      iv. adjust I-time using a reference range
      v. leave all other settings at machine defaults unless one of these considerations applies:

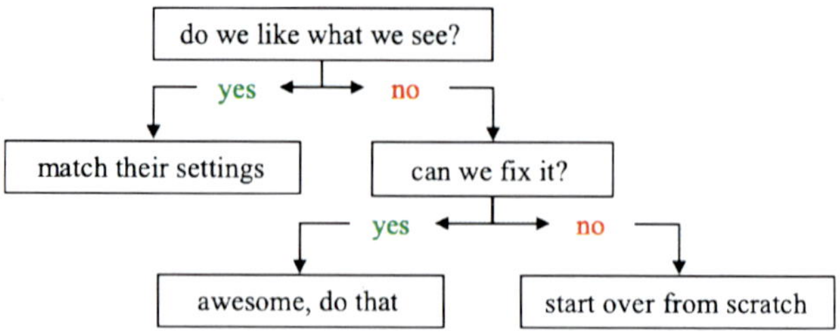

age description	age (years)	RR	I-time (s)
infant	.083 (1 month) – 1	30 – 53	0.3 – 0.7
toddler	1 – 2	22 – 37	0.4 – 0.9
preschooler	3 – 5	22 – 28	0.5 – 0.9
school-aged child	6 – 7	18 – 25	0.6 – 1.1
big kids	8 – 9	17 – 25	0.6 – 1.2
preadolescent	10 – 12	14 – 23	0.7 – 1.4
adolescent	12 – 15	12 – 20	0.8 – 1.7
adult	16 and up	12 – 20	0.8 – 1.7

strategy	things to do
obstruction	decrease I:E ratio (1:≥5) by decreasing rate (and maybe I-time also), then titrate tidal volume (or pressure control) up to maintain minute volume as able; consider less PEEP
hypotension	limit PEEP; increase tidal volume and then decrease rate to maintain minute volume
acidosis	use high end of tidal volume (8ml/kg IBW); increase rate: pre-intubation rate, to get prior/goal $EtCO_2$, or double normal value
lung injury	higher PEEP

3. initiate ventilation (clamp tube if concerned with de-recruitment)

II. Address the Three Big Things

parameter	assessment	normal	actions
oxygenation	SpO_2	93-99%	*low:* consider position & suction, increase FiO_2, increase PEEP, increase I-time, consider pathophysiology/ medications, think V/Q mismatch *high:* decrease FiO_2 unless contraindicated (i.e. pregnancy, anemia, shock, etc.)
ventilation	$EtCO_2$	35-45mmHg (low end for TBI)	*any abnormal value:* consider etiology &/ or patient compensation for acid-base imbalance (may be appropriate) *low:* consider perfusion status; decrease rate, then decrease tidal volume *high:* increase tidal volume (monitor plateau pressure), then increase rate; consider permissive hypercapnia
	MV	≈ 100ml/kg/min (2x with acidosis)	*low:* increase tidal volume (monitor plateau pressure), then increase rate; consider permissive hypercapnia *high:* decrease rate, then decrease tidal volume; consider SIMV
comfort	RASS, ANVPS	at provider discretion	*extreme end:* analgesia & sedation *fine tuning:* address triggers, lengthen inspiratory time (I:E ratio closer to 1:1), trial different mode/ control (and increase pressure support in SIMV)

III. Keep Things Going

1. set (and troubleshoot) all alarms
2. consider pressures (every time vitals get reassessed)

parameter	normal	actions
peak inspiratory pressure	$<35\text{cmH}_2\text{O}$	consider potential causes (**lung** and **airway issues**), check plateau pressure decrease tidal volume (or pressure control)
plateau pressure	$<30\text{cmH}_2\text{O}$	consider potential causes (**lung issues**) decrease tidal volume (or pressure control)
AutoPEEP	none	decrease I:E ratio/ extend expiratory time (lower rate, shorter inspiratory time) consider triggering, trial volume control if in pressure control, adjust PEEP disconnect circuit to allow exhalation
driving pressure	$<15\text{cmH}_2\text{O}$	decrease tidal volume or pressure control consider more PEEP and permissive hypercapnia consider recruitment maneuvers
mean airway pressure	not applicable	monitor for trends and investigate further

3. make adjustments moving forward

strategy	things to do
general stuff	if oxygenation is all good, go down on FiO_2 (maybe all the way to 0.40) and reevaluate consider increasing tidal volume to safe plateau pressure and acceptable driving pressure
obstruction	use drugs (in-line neb treatment, consider Ketamine for analgesia/ sedation, etc.) ensure no AutoPEEP develops if hypercapnia develops and/ or no AutoPEEP noted, consider moving towards normal I:E ratio
hypotension	use caution with PEEP to improve oxygenation consider fluid and/ or pressors if perfusion improves, consider working towards normal settings to avoid higher pressures
acidosis	maintain increased minute volume goal (minimum 200ml/kg/min) also consider Winter's Formula to guide treatment
lung injury	consider titrating tidal volume down to 5ml/kg, then 4ml/kg to maintain driving pressure $<15\text{cmH}_2\text{O}$ increase PEEP to maximize oxygenation, consider stepwise approach consider recruitment maneuver if hypoxia persists

IV. Fix Problems When They Come Up

acute deterioration: what to do!?

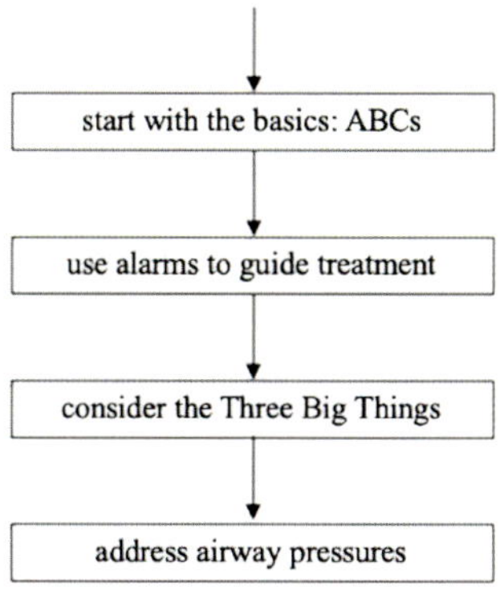

lung issues

- abdominal distention/ ascites → reposition or elevate head of bed
- atelectasis → recruit some alveoli (via PEEP and/or recruitment maneuvers)
- AutoPEEP → decrease I:E ratio, trial volume control, maybe adjust PEEP, disconnect circuit
- chest wall burn → escharotomy
- pneumonia → utilize PEEP to displace fluid
- pneumothorax → remove from vent; needle decompression, chest tube, or finger thoracotomy
- pulmonary contusion → consider lung injury strategy
- pulmonary edema → utilize PEEP to displace fluid
- tube migration → deflate cuff, pull back, re-inflate

airway issues

- aspiration → suction (prevent further aspiration), consider lung injury strategy
- bronchospasm → fix with drugs, implement obstruction strategy
- endotracheal tube occlusion → address comfort (biting), swap tube (something stuck)
- secretions → suction

Suggestions for Further Study

Just some guidance based on what kind of medium someone is looking for. This is not an exhaustive list, but just some places to start for getting better at the management of vented patients. Also recognize that each of these references has way more to offer than just the specific content linked, browse them all for more intel on many of the things we've discussed in this manual.

audio/ podcast

EMCrit Dominating the Vent Series

FlightBridgeED Vent Series

video, vent specific

Strong Medicine Series on Mechanical Ventilation

Hospitalista Series on Mechanical Ventilation

video, physiology

Ninja Nerd Science, section on Respiratory

Khan Academy, section on Advanced Respiratory System Physiology

text, web-based

Deranged Physiology, section on Respiratory

RebelEM, Simplifying Mechanical Ventilation

text, free eBook

Principles and Practices of Mechanical Ventilation by Martin J. Tobin (3rd edition)

text, books to buy

Ventilator Management: A Pre-Hospital Perspective by Eric Bauer

Vent Hero: Advanced Transport Ventilator Management by Charles Swearingen

a – arterial; **A** – alveolar; **cmH₂O** – centimeters of water; **FiO₂** – fraction of inspired oxygen; **mmHg** – millimeters of mercury; **PAO₂** – partial pressure of alveolar oxygen; **PaO₂** – partial pressure of arterial oxygen

Appendix

Alveolar Gas Equation

The alveolar gas equation allows us to calculate the partial pressure of oxygen in the alveoli in a given set of circumstances. We used this equation to get values listed in some of the graphics throughout this manual:

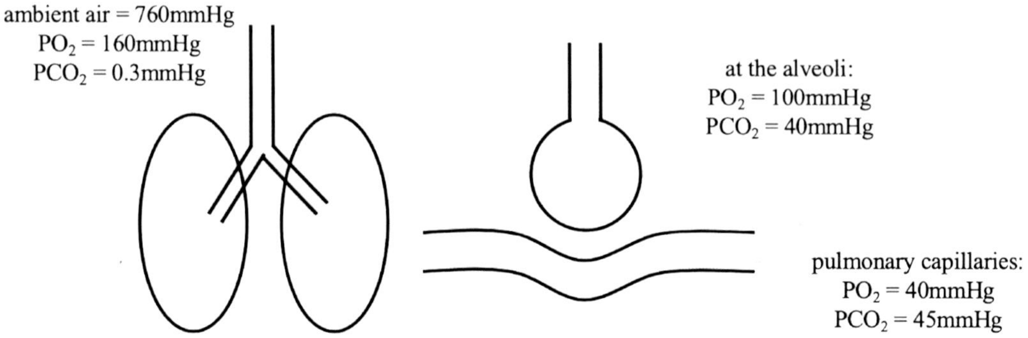

because there is an open system between the ambient air and the alveoli, the overall pressure at the alveoli is also 760mmHg at baseline, however the partial pressures of the components are different along the way

The equation goes like this:[304]

$$PAO_2 = FiO_2(P_{atm} - P_{water}) - (PaCO_2/RespQ)$$

PAO_2 is partial pressure of alveolar oxygen
FiO_2 is fraction of inspired oxygen, 0.21 for ambient air
P_{atm} is atmospheric pressure
P_{water} is partial pressure of water vapor at the alveoli, 47mmHg at sea level
$PaCO_2$ is as measured by blood gas (or approximated from $EtCO_2$), we'll say 40mmHg
RespQ is respiratory quotient and is assumed to be 0.8[305]

given that RespQ = 0.8, we sometimes see the equation simplified as so:

$$PAO_2 = FiO_2(P_{atm} - P_{water}) - 1.25(PaCO_2)$$

and since P_{atm}, P_{water}, and $PaCO_2$ are all held constant in our thought experiments:

$$PAO_2 = FiO_2(760 - 47) - 50$$

[304] Yartsev, 2019 – He's got a good graphic that shows the alveolar gas equation with all parts labeled, maybe makes a bit more sense to the visual learners than how it is represented here

[305] Patel & Bhardwaj, 2018 – These guys describe the details behind this respiratory quotient idea; maybe not relevant to our discussion of vent stuff, but good nerdy details for those who want more (another option would be to find an exercise physiology textbook, likely to be some good stuff there)

P_{atm} – atmospheric pressure; **PCO_2** – partial pressure of carbon dioxide; **PEEP** – positive end-expiratory pressure; **PO_2** – partial pressure of oxygen; **RespQ** – respiratory quotient

$$PAO_2 = FiO_2(713) - 50$$

but back to our original equation:

$$PAO_2 = FiO_2(P_{atm} - P_{water}) - (PaCO_2/RespQ)$$
$$PAO_2 = 0.21(760 - 47) - (40/0.8)$$
$$PAO_2 \approx 100mmHg$$

other iterations of the alveolar gas equation that we demonstrated in the manual are shown here:

PAO_2 at 100% or FiO_2 1.0 (no PEEP)

$$PAO_2 = FiO_2(760 - 47) - 50$$
$$PAO_2 = 663mmHg$$

PAO_2 with 5cm PEEP (room air)[306]

$$PAO_2 = FiO_2(760\ (+\ 4) - 47) - 50$$
$$PAO_2 \approx 101mmHg$$

So we can use the alveolar gas equation to solve algebra problems in an effort to show how things like **Fraction of Inspired Oxygen** and **Positive End-Expiratory Pressure** affect PAO_2. And then if we know how much oxygen should be getting to the alveoli and can measure how much oxygen made it into the arteries (PaO_2 from a blood gas), then maybe we can understand something about the efficacy of that exchange. To say it another way, the idea is that we can use values for PAO_2 and PaO_2 to inform us on what is going on with a patient in reference to the movement of oxygen from the input of our vent system into the bloodstream. Values like A-a Gradient and a/A Ratio attempt to do just that. Now there are some limitations to both of these values and their application may be limited in the transport setting, so we won't get into the details here.[307]

[306] Just a friendly reminder that $5cmH_2O$ is roughly 4mmHg, see chart in **Measuring Pressures**

[307] Strong, 2014; Yartsev, 2019 – The first is a video that explains A-a gradient; the second is an articles that discusses these types of measurements and identifies issues with their application to clinical practice

ARDS – acute respiratory distress syndrome; **cmH₂O** – centimeters of water; **EtCO₂** – end-tidal carbon dioxide; **FeCO₂** – fraction of exhaled CO₂; **IBW** – ideal body weight; **kg** – kilogram; **L** – liter; **min** – minute; **ml** – milliliter; **mmHg** – millimeters of mercury; **MV** – minute volume

Mechanical Dead Space

In order to determine the effect of mechanical dead space, we first need to know how much volume each of the extra components takes up. This varies a lot depending on which specific devices we use and can be found on product labels, but we'll just generalize it here:

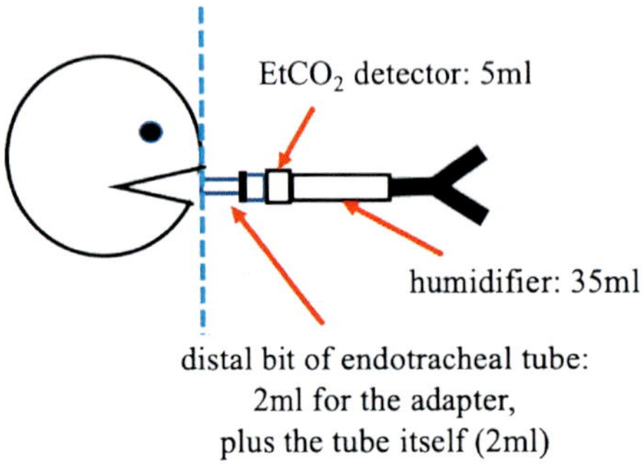

other potential things
in-line suction contraption/ angle: 5ml
flexible angle adapters: 10ml
filter: 50ml or more!

total estimate: 50ml
(excluding the filter, since we often put it elsewhere)

Let's say we want to figure out to what effect 50ml of added **Dead Space** impacts **Ventilation** in our patients. Now this gets a little weird and the math takes a few leaps of faith along the way, but let's follow along and then compare what we come up with to data after the fact. Also, note that we are going to introduce a few new ideas here and that we will get more into those in the very next section:[308]

assume a patient of 65kg IBW
being ventilated at TV 6ml/kg (390ml) and RR of 17
MV calculated = 6630ml/min

now we already said a few things about this:
alveolar TV = TV – anatomic dead space
and this dead space is approximately 1/3 of TV
so alveolar TV = 260ml
VA = RR x alveolar TV
in this case VA = 4420ml/min

and if we add 50ml more of dead space into the situation
alveolar TV = TV – anatomic dead space – mechanical dead space
so alveolar TV = 210ml
VA = RR x (alveolar TV – mechanical dead space)
in this case VA = 3570ml/min

[308] And to review these ideas: **Ideal Body Weight**, **Tidal Volume**, **Respiratory Rate**, and **Minute Volume**

OK – alright; **$PaCO_2$** – partial pressure of arterial CO_2; **$PACO_2$** – partial pressure of alveolar CO_2; **P_{atm}** – atmospheric pressure; **$PECO_2$** – mean partial pressure of exhaled CO_2; **pH** – power of hydrogen; **P_{water}** – partial pressure of water vapor; **RR** – respiratory rate; **TV** – tidal volume; **VA** – alveolar minute volume; **V_D** – dead space

We already know that there can be a discrepancy between these two versions of alveolar minute volume, the one with mechanical dead space left out and the one with it included. But now let's consider the idea that the amount of carbon dioxide produced per minute doesn't change from case to case, rather it's simply the case that less of that of it gets exhaled. So how much carbon dioxide gets left behind in the system what and kind of effect does that have on the body? To answer the first question, let's look at the following relationship:

$$\frac{V_D}{TV} = \frac{EtCO_2 - PECO_2}{EtCO_2}$$

Now there are two versions of this formula that use $PACO_2$ and $PaCO_2$ rather than $EtCO_2$, but it has been proposed that this representation might be of value in calculating dead space in practice.[309] So simply for the sake of this example, we will go with that. Now that $PECO_2$ value is something we haven't discussed yet; it is the mean partial pressure of carbon dioxide during exhalation. A normal value is around 30mmHg and it could also be calculated based on the idea that a normal fraction of expired carbon dioxide ($FeCO_2$) is about 4%:[310]

$$PECO_2 = FeCO_2\,(P_{atm} - P_{water})$$
$$PECO_2 = 4\%\,(760\text{mmHg} - 47\text{mmHg})$$
$$PECO_2 \approx 28.5$$

now if we use that value and the previous equation,
we can solve for an expected $EtCO_2$ in either of the dead space cases in question

only anatomic dead space:

$$\frac{130}{390} = \frac{EtCO_2 - 28.5}{EtCO_2}$$
$$EtCO_2 \approx 43$$

with mechanical dead space added in:

$$\frac{180}{390} = \frac{EtCO_2 - 28.5}{EtCO_2}$$
$$EtCO_2 \approx 53$$

---

309 Siobal, 2016 – This is a theoretical thing and would require further experimentation, but it serves the purpose of showing to what extent dead space might impact quantitative measures of $EtCO_2$, with all other things being equal

310 ScyMed, 2018 – Good reference for calculations and normal values for all things physiology

ARDS – acute respiratory distress syndrome; **cmH₂O** – centimeters of water; **EtCO₂** – end-tidal carbon dioxide; **FeCO₂** – fraction of exhaled CO₂; **IBW** – ideal body weight; **kg** – kilogram; **L** – liter; **min** – minute; **ml** – milliliter; **mmHg** – millimeters of mercury; **MV** – minute volume

Now a difference in $EtCO_2$ of 10mmHg doesn't necessarily mean that a corresponding quantity of carbon dioxide remains in the blood and impacts the body. The purpose of this exercise was simply to show that the potential exists for a buildup of carbon dioxide in the alveoli. In the transport setting where $EtCO_2$ monitoring is routinely used to assess ventilation, we would simply increase **Minute Volume** to bring that second value into a normal range. But let's suspend that idea for just a moment longer and consider what impact this might have if we failed to do that. Researchers looked at this very problem and determined that removing 115ml of dead space from a circuit resulted in a decrease in $PaCO_2$ of 11mmHg and an increase of pH from 7.30 to 7.38.[311] Furthermore, they were able to do that with less minute volume. Now this was in patients with ARDS in which one of our concerns is the amount of air needed to maintain ventilation and consequences of that air on the patient's pulmonary system, but the findings are pretty significant.

Back to our discussion and application to the transport setting: we said just a moment ago that we could potentially avoid this increased carbon dioxide retention by monitoring $EtCO_2$ and increasing minute volume to accommodate, but the truth is that doing so isn't always a benign thing. Going up on **Tidal Volume** or **Pressure Control** will increase pressure (**Plateau Pressure** and **Driving Pressure**), while going up on **Respiratory Rate** has the potential to cause discomfort and increase that percentage of time at decreased preload (%TaDP) concept.[312] If we can promote carbon dioxide removal while simultaneously avoiding all of those things, this seems like a pretty good reason to be conscious of adding unnecessary things into the vent circuit whenever possible.

[311] Hinkson & friends, 2006 – Even though the study had a small sample size, the findings support that support this idea of limiting mechanical dead space

[312] Refer back to **Comfort** and **Hypotension** to review these idea

OK – alright; **$PaCO_2$** – partial pressure of arterial CO_2; **$PACO_2$** – partial pressure of alveolar CO_2; **P_{atm}** – atmospheric pressure; **$PECO_2$** – mean partial pressure of exhaled CO_2; **pH** – power of hydrogen; **P_{water}** – partial pressure of water vapor; **RR** – respiratory rate; **TV** – tidal volume; **$\dot{V}A$** – alveolar minute volume; **V_D** – dead space

One last thing about all of this with regards to pediatrics and volume control ventilation. We mentioned way back when that it's OK if our calculated minute volume is larger than our goal minute volume because of some complications posed by dead space.[313] We want to revisit that to show why that is and how we can mitigate it all. The example was a 4-year-old kid of 18kg:

TV = 6 – 8ml/kg IBW
TV = 6 – 8ml/kg x 18kg
TV = 108 – 144ml

MV goal = 100ml/kg IBW/min
MV goal = 1800ml/min
MV goal = 1.8L/min

MV calculated = RR x TV
MV calculated = (20 – 28)/min x (108 – 144)ml
MV calculated = 2160– 4032ml/min
MV calculated ≈ 2.2 – 4L/min

Just as with the adult patient, we have anatomic dead space that is always there and then mechanical dead space that we add in. But we never did consider that the vent tubing itself has some flex to it. If we look closely at the label of our vent tubing, it may say something like "compliance 0.0008L/cmH_2O." So let's take that hypothetical example and run with it:

we'll go with a TV of 6ml/kg (108ml) and a RR of 24
MV calculated = 2592ml/min
VA = RR x (TV – dead space)

to summarize all the dead space components:
we know we have about 36ml (1/3 of TV) anatomic dead space
let's say 20ml of mechanical because we have a pedi humidifier and EtCO_2 detector
and let's assume a driving pressure of 12cmH_2O to get to our TV goal
0.0008L/cmH_2O x 12cmH_2O ≈ 10ml
total dead space = 36ml + 20ml + 10ml
total dead space = 66ml

VA = 24/min x (108ml – 66ml)
VA = 1008ml/min

313 We first mentioned this consideration (of dead space with pediatric patients) in **A General Vent Strategy**

ARDS – acute respiratory distress syndrome; **cmH_2O** – centimeters of water; **$EtCO_2$** – end-tidal carbon dioxide; **$FeCO_2$** – fraction of exhaled CO_2; **IBW** – ideal body weight; **kg** – kilogram; **L** – liter; **min** – minute; **ml** – milliliter; **mmHg** – millimeters of mercury; **MV** – minute volume

Now in this case the alveolar minute volume is low (minute volume goal was 1.8L/min), but we could then look at exhaled tidal volume and $EtCO_2$ to titrate up to an appropriate level. But what if this had been a 10kg two-year-old?

TV 6ml/kg = 60ml
total dead space = 66ml
which mathematically means no actual ventilation!

Just to be clear, this isn't completely the case. As tidal volume decreases we likely get less anatomic dead space as airway structures don't flex and expand as they normally would with the delivery of normal-sized breaths. We mentioned before that we assume dead space is constant when going up on tidal volume, but there is some variation here and it is most notable the extreme end of low.[314] Knowing to what degree this type of thing happens isn't generally possible in transport, but the takeaway point still stands – be sure to consider these things when ventilating in volume control with small volumes.

One last thing to consider is the idea that if we are using uncuffed endotracheal tubes with our kids, some tidal volume may get lost as air moves back past the tube to the oropharynx.[315] So the moral of the story here is that we should either ventilate these patients in pressure control (to bypass this vent circuit stretch dead space concept) or start at a higher end of normal tidal volume and be ready to quickly go up on minute volume as soon as initiating ventilation in volume control (based on exhaled tidal volume and $EtCO_2$). As we said before, there is no right or wrong to this, so long as we know the consequences and correct actions associated with whatever choice we make.

[314] Yartsev, 2019 – We mentioned this idea that dead space does vary with tidal volume delivered back in both **Dead Space** and **Ventilation**; this same article also explains that this relationship is not constant across a body's capacity and that there seems to be less dead space with smaller tidal volumes
[315] Chambers & friends, 2017 – For more information on cuffed versus uncuffed tubes with pediatrics, take a look at this paper

I:E – inspiratory to expiratory; **I-time** – inspiratory time; **PALS** – Pediatric Advanced Life Support; **RR** – respiratory rate; **s** – second

Age-Based Settings

In an effort to make recommendations about vent settings for specific age groups, specifically **Respiratory Rate** and **Inspiratory Time**, here's how the process went:

1. Make assumptions:
    a. Normal Respiratory Rates as outlined by PALS are good enough to work with
    b. Normal respiratory rate range for an adult is 12-20 (cited in many, many sources)
    c. A normal I:E ratio at rest and spontaneous respiration is 1:2, but we often work with a ratio of 1:3 for vented patients[316]

2. Fill the gaps in the PALS Normal Respiratory Rates data set:
    a. What gaps?[317]

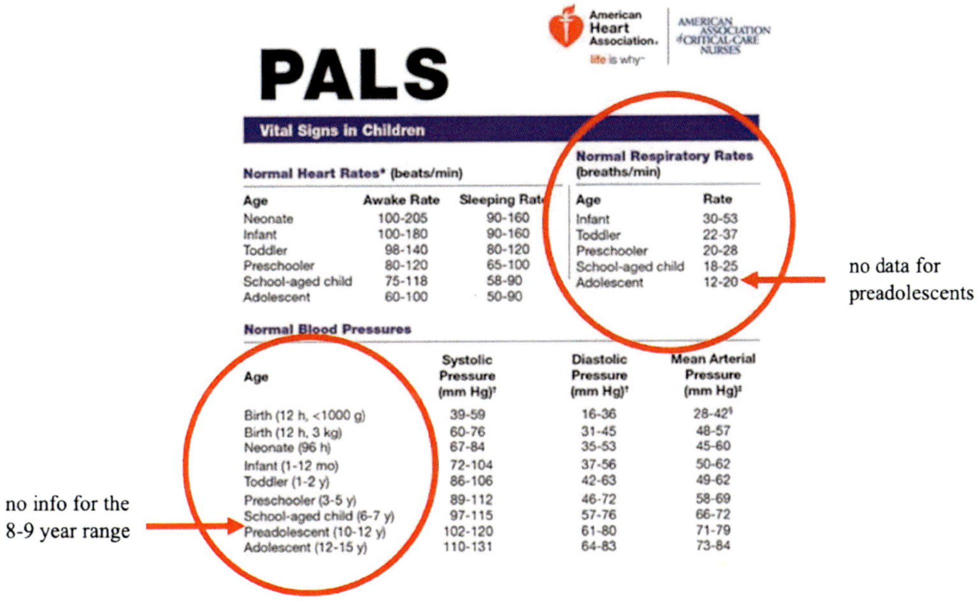

Normal Heart Rates* (beats/min)

Age	Awake Rate	Sleeping Rate
Neonate	100-205	90-160
Infant	100-180	90-160
Toddler	98-140	80-120
Preschooler	80-120	65-100
School-aged child	75-118	58-90
Adolescent	60-100	50-90

Normal Respiratory Rates (breaths/min)

Age	Rate
Infant	30-53
Toddler	22-37
Preschooler	20-28
School-aged child	18-25
Adolescent	12-20

Normal Blood Pressures

Age	Systolic Pressure (mm Hg)†	Diastolic Pressure (mm Hg)†	Mean Arterial Pressure (mm Hg)‡
Birth (12 h, <1000 g)	39-59	16-36	28-42§
Birth (12 h, 3 kg)	60-76	31-45	48-57
Neonate (96 h)	67-84	35-53	45-60
Infant (1-12 mo)	72-104	37-56	50-62
Toddler (1-2 y)	86-106	42-63	49-62
Preschooler (3-5 y)	89-112	46-72	58-69
School-aged child (6-7 y)	97-115	57-76	66-72
Preadolescent (10-12 y)	102-120	61-80	71-79
Adolescent (12-15 y)	110-131	64-83	73-84

---

[316] And this may be by convention of leaving inspiratory time set at a given value, not necessarily because that's the thing we ought to be doing; but regardless, we'll get a range of possible values using both 1:2 and 1:3

[317] American Heart Association, 2016 (image) – And we said already (section on **Respiratory Rate**) that we chose to use these values not because they are intended for use with vent management, but because they represent normal values by age and are from a reference that most of us are familiar with and have access to

I:E – inspiratory to expiratory; **I-time** – inspiratory time; **PALS** – Pediatric Advanced Life Support; **RR** – respiratory rate; **s** – second

b. Plot the existing data using both high and low ends of rate by age, make charts, then add lines of best fit:

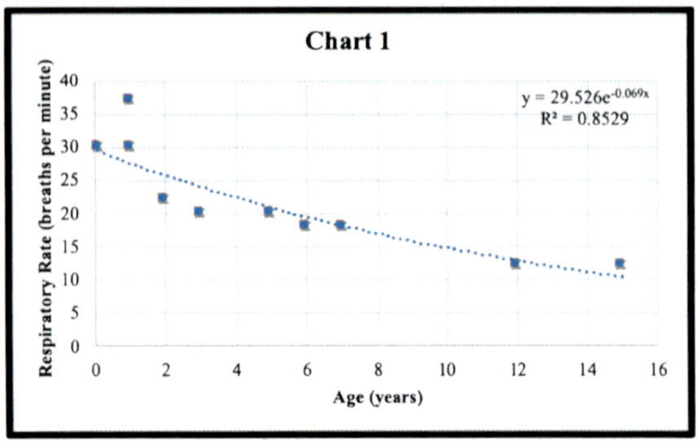

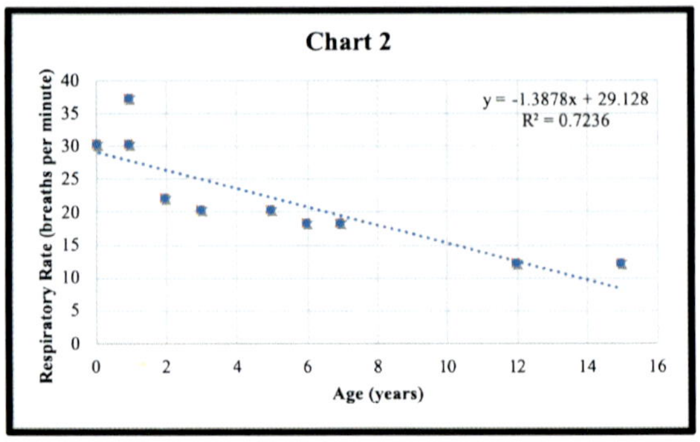

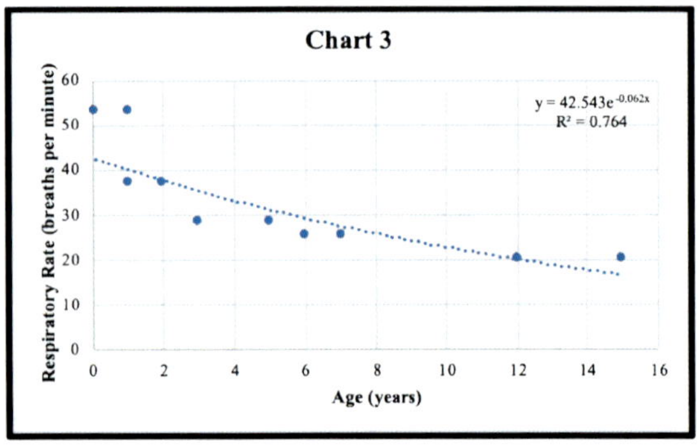

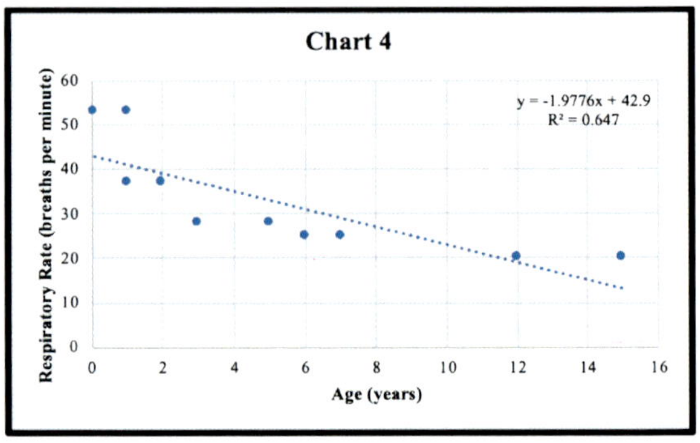

c. Using the better fits (exponential regression), solve for the missing data points in the PALS chart, then add those values into a new chart (noted in blue):

age description	age (years)	rate
infant	.083 (1 month) – 1	30 – 53
toddler	1 – 2	22 – 37
preschooler	3 – 5	20 – 28
school-aged child	6 – 7	18 – 25
big kids	8 – 9	17 – 25[318]
preadolescent	10 – 12	14 – 23
adolescent	12 – 15	12 – 20
adult	16 and up	12 – 20

[318] Range here was calculated to be 17-26, but we went with 25 since range for school-aged child was to a max of 25 – this was an arbitrary decision, but makes the final product flow a bit better

I:E – inspiratory to expiratory; **I-time** – inspiratory time; **PALS** – Pediatric Advanced Life Support; **RR** – respiratory rate; **s** – second

3. Do a lot of calculations (for inspiratory times):

60s ÷ RR = time per each respiratory cycle
ex. for adult (low end RR): 60 ÷ 12 = 5s
ex. for adult (high end RR): 60 ÷ 20 = 3s

I-time = time per each respiratory cycle ÷ number of parts in that cycle
ex. for adult (low end RR, 1:2): 5s ÷ 3 ≈ 1.7
ex. for adult (high end RR, 1:3): 5s ÷ 4 ≈ 0.8

therefore I-time range for adults is 0.8 – 1.7s

4. Put all the data into a chart:

age description	**age (years)**	**rate**	**I-time (s)**
infant	.083 (1 month) – 1	30 – 53	0.3 – 0.7
toddler	1 – 2	22 – 37	0.4 – 0.9
preschooler	3 – 5	22 – 28	0.5 – 0.9
school-aged child	6 – 7	18 – 25	0.6 – 1.1
big kids	8 – 9	17 – 25	0.6 – 1.2
preadolescent	10 – 12	14 – 23	0.7 – 1.4
adolescent	12 – 15	12 – 20	0.8 – 1.7
adult	16 and up	12 – 20	0.8 – 1.7

I-time – inspiratory time; **kg** – kilogram; **ml** – milliliter; **min** – minute; **MV** – minute volume; **OK** – alright; P_{aw} – mean airway pressure

Hypotension Strategy Math

In the section where we outlined the **Hypotension** strategy, we introduced a concept which we called percentage of time at decreased preload (%TaDP). The idea was that if we decrease the overall amount of time spent pushing air into the system above our set **Positive End-Expiratory Pressure** (i.e. inspiration) then we can mitigate the exacerbation of a hypotensive state. The result was a strategy that included a shorter **Inspiratory Time**, higher **Tidal Volume**, and lower **Respiratory Rate**. We also mentioned that there are other rationales for this strategy: less **Dead Space** and lower **Mean Airway Pressure**. We are going to calculate these differences here just to give some more legitimacy to the argument.

But before we get there, one other thing to mention. PEEP is also a contributing factor to hypotension in the susceptible patient, so we want to keep that to a minimum. While it may seem like a good idea to drop PEEP to zero in the hypotensive patient (especially in light of the mean airway pressure calculations we'll show in just a moment), recognize that **Oxygenation** is also super important and PEEP is one of our tools to maintain that. Other specific benefits of PEEP that'd we'd like to maintain in these patients include ease of triggering spontaneous breaths and alveolar recruitment. Last thing: the positive-pressure ventilation/ PEEP → decreased preload → decreased cardiac output sequence of events can be mitigated by fluid resuscitation.[319]

Moving forward, recognize that is totally OK to drop PEEP all the way to zero if need be, but there may be consequences and there may be other relatively simple strategies (i.e. fluids and other vent changes) to mitigate the negative consequences while maintaining the benefits. It's also just fine to drop PEEP to zero in an emergency, then work back up to a beneficial level after the acute threat has passed and other interventions have been put into place. Vent management is dynamic and we can adjust strategy as we move forward with patient care. So while we are going to show how eliminating PEEP can significantly reduce mean airway pressure, which theoretically lessens the negative consequences of positive-pressure ventilation, just know that there are multiple variables involved in this practice.

[319] We mentioned this sequence of events and how to mitigate it with fluids way back in **How is Positive-Pressure Ventilation Different?**

PEEP – positive end-expiratory pressure; **PIP** – peak inspiratory pressure; **s** – second; **T_{total}** – amount of time per breath; **V̇A** – alveolar minute volume

Now for the math, starting with how the lower rate, higher tidal volume strategy decreases dead space. Let's assume another 65kg patient and see how it looks. We've shown the calculations here working from the assumption that anatomic dead space doesn't change with tidal volume, but recognize that this idea is based on a number of factors and may not be the case for all situations:[320]

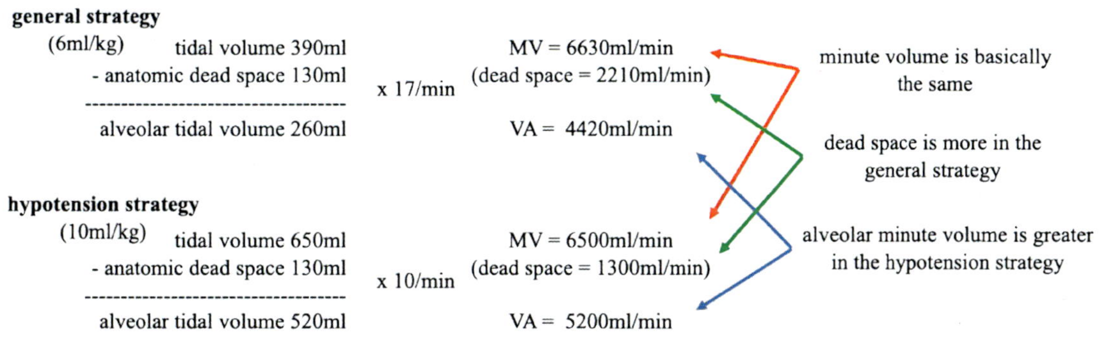

This demonstrates the concept that in the hypotensive strategy we push less wasted air into the system. We already know that positive pressure, whether in the form of a breath being delivered or PEEP, has potential negative consequences, so if we eliminate any part of that (i.e. reduce dead space) while maintaining ventilation then our patient is better off. To say it another way, we want to try to make use (in the form of alveolar minute volume) of as much of the total air (minute volume) that we put into the system in an effort to eliminate pushing air in unnecessarily (dead space).

The next concept to discuss is mean airway pressure. The airways and lungs live inside the thoracic cavity, so if we put pressure into the respiratory system then we see changes to pressure in the thoracic cavity. The idea is that mean airway pressure directly correlates with a concept called intrathoracic pressure and intrathoracic pressure, in turn, is the thing that causes all those hemodynamic changes associated with positive-pressure ventilation.[321] Now it gets exponentially more complex than that, as pressure at specific components within that thoracic cavity, all of which are tied to hemodynamic function, vary significantly (in terms of influence on function, not necessarily quantitatively), but the simple interpretation of the idea is that pressure we put in via the vent can disrupt hemodynamic function and result in less cardiac output.[322] So theoretically, if we limit mean airway pressure we can minimize these potential negative consequences.

Mean airway pressure is normally measured by the vent itself, but there is a formula to estimate it using values for inspiratory time, **Peak Inspiratory Pressure**, and PEEP (and also T_{total}, which is the amount of time per breath or 60s ÷ respiratory rate):

$$P_{aw} = 0.5 \times (PIP - PEEP) \times (I\text{-}time/T_{total}) + PEEP$$

[320] Yartsev, 2019 – To say it another way, this advantage that we calculate out is the best case scenario; we talked about this in **Ventilation** and referenced this same article then; also refer back to **A General Vent Strategy** to review that idea
[321] Chiefetz, 2014; Luecke & Pelosi, 2005 – Both articles get into the details of intrathoracic pressure related to positive-pressure ventilation and the many interactions and consequences involved

I-time – inspiratory time; **kg** – kilogram; **ml** – milliliter; **min** – minute; **MV** – minute volume; **OK** – alright; P_{aw} – mean airway pressure

Using this formula, we built a spreadsheet of possible mean airway pressure (P_{aw}) data points for each strategy with different values for peak inspiratory pressure (PIP) and PEEP. And just to clarify, this is with an inspiratory time of 1.0s in both cases and a rate of 17 per the general strategy:

general strategy							
P_{aw}		PIP					
		10	15	20	25	30	35
PEEP	0	1.42	2.13	2.83	3.54	4.25	4.96
	1	2.28	2.98	3.69	4.40	5.11	5.82
	2	3.13	3.84	4.55	5.26	5.97	6.68
	3	3.99	4.70	5.41	6.12	6.83	7.53
	4	4.85	5.56	6.27	6.98	7.68	8.39
	5	5.71	6.42	7.13	7.83	8.54	9.25
	6	6.57	7.28	7.98	8.69	9.40	10.1

hypotensive strategy							
P_{aw}		PIP					
		10	15	20	25	30	35
PEEP	0	0.67	1.00	1.33	1.67	2.00	2.33
	1	1.60	1.93	2.27	2.60	2.93	3.27
	2	2.53	2.87	3.20	3.53	3.87	4.20
	3	3.47	3.80	4.13	4.47	4.80	5.13
	4	4.40	4.73	5.07	5.40	5.73	6.07
	5	5.33	5.67	6.00	6.33	6.67	7.00
	6	6.27	6.60	6.93	7.27	7.60	7.93

Barring the most drastic possible scenario (excellent **Compliance** and very low peak pressure) per the general strategy, poor compliance and high peak pressure with transition to the hypotensive strategy; paired with keeping PEEP constant), we can see that the hypotensive strategy tends to give lower numbers for mean airway pressure. While it is likely that overall compliance will decrease and thus peak inspiratory pressure will increase as we move from left to right (due to higher tidal volume with the hypotensive strategy), guesstimating to what degree that will happen seems unfair without actual experimental data. There may also be a mathematical model based on this idea that could identify cases where mean airway pressure isn't actually decreased with the hypotensive strategy, but given that this is just one of three reasons to use the strategy (the other two being lower percentage of time at decreased preload and less dead space), it seems OK for now.

Just to demonstrate an arbitrary example, if we had a patient vented per the general strategy with a peak inspiratory pressure of 20 and transitioned them to the hypotensive strategy and ended up with a peak pressure of 30, we'd get a drop in mean airway pressure:

general strategy							
P_{aw}		PIP					
		10	15	20	25	30	35
PEEP	0	1.42	2.13	2.83	3.54	4.25	4.96
	1	2.28	2.98	3.69	4.40	5.11	5.82
	2	3.13	3.84	4.55	5.26	5.97	6.68
	3	3.99	4.70	5.41	6.12	6.83	7.53
	4	4.85	5.56	6.27	6.98	7.68	8.39
	5	5.71	6.42	7.13	7.83	8.54	9.25
	6	6.57	7.28	7.98	8.69	9.40	10.1

hypotensive strategy							
P_{aw}		PIP					
		10	15	20	25	30	35
PEEP	0	0.67	1.00	1.33	1.67	2.00	2.33
	1	1.60	1.93	2.27	2.60	2.93	3.27
	2	2.53	2.87	3.20	3.53	3.87	4.20
	3	3.47	3.80	4.13	4.47	4.80	5.13
	4	4.40	4.73	5.07	5.40	5.73	6.07
	5	5.33	5.67	6.00	6.33	6.67	7.00
	6	6.27	6.60	6.93	7.27	7.60	7.93

At this point there are no experimental data (at least that we are aware of) to show to what extent this type of thing has on cardiac output or other parameters of hemodynamic function, but given the logical sequence of events that we already outlined it seems like a step in the right direction for the hypotensive patient or one at risk for becoming so.

PEEP – positive end-expiratory pressure; **PIP** – peak inspiratory pressure; **s** – second; **T_{total}** – amount of time per breath; **$\dot{V}A$** – alveolar minute volume

Just to summarize things for this section: the hypotensive strategy includes shorter inspiratory time, increased tidal volume, lower respiratory rate, and keeping PEEP to the lowest level needed to maintain oxygenation. We discussed the idea of percentage of decreased preload (%TaDP) back in the section on hypotension and then we added to that just now the idea that this approach results in both less dead space and a generally lower mean airway pressure. And while PEEP is a major contributor to mean airway pressure, it also serves to maintain oxygenation; this means we ought to use caution in titrating it all the down to zero.

A Personal Reflection

When I started putting this all together I thought I knew a fair amount about vents. At least I thought I knew enough to effectively manage patients in transport and that my comprehension of it all was adequate to simplify it for others. Turns out I still had (and have!) a long way to go. In spite of this realization, the process of putting in all down in words and images has helped me learn way more than I thought I would've needed to. And I think this final product will satisfactorily help others achieve a better understanding of vents with the ultimate outcome being improved care for the patients we move around.

Another thing that came up in this process was an awareness of how choice of language can contribute to a project like this. One could say that I have a baseline aversion to formality and convention. My preferred venue for this chat about vents would've been a backyard patio with beer in hand. My initial drafts reflected this a bit more at the potential cost of alienating readers. I've tried to find a balance, so we'll see how that turns out. And mad props to both Ben and Bruce for being frank with me about that.

Carrying on with that idea, Ben made the point that my readers are likely professionals in a niche setting and, because of that, it may help to reference certain concepts that all of us ought to keep hidden away in the back of our collective brain. For example, I was reluctant to include references to both gas laws and the oxyhemoglobin dissociation curve, as I didn't want to fall into the trap of putting out content specific for test takers or to be seen as taking away from really good material that's already out there. But the point was not lost on me that there is, in fact, a middle ground, so I've tried to accommodate those ideas.

I've also come to realize that organizing thoughts coherently is quite a chore. I wanted a sequential progression of concepts from start to finish, but also a format that allows for quick referencing and jumping between sections. Thanks to Dan for pointing out that something as simple as a legend at the top of each page can help significantly with this process. And then within that overall framework there were countless explanations that got erased and then rewritten multiple times. Same goes for those graphics I used to try and replace words. Bruce, I appreciate your feedback on that front and am sure that things will be clearer for folks because of it.

And lastly, thanks to Chris for giving in to my persistent bullying and for reviewing the last draft from start to finish. He talked me into keeping it simple and spelling things out longhand, provided valuable insight on a number of the graphics, and asked good questions about how some of these theoretical concepts actually play out in practice. And while we didn't have a backyard patio for our vent book banter, we made the best of the situation and used the rooftop of his New York City apartment to hash all these ideas out.

The goal from the beginning was that this is to be an ongoing project. I'm sure there are errors and misunderstandings hiding in plain sight, but that's all part of the learning process. If you come across something that needs attention or even if you just want to get involved in the next version, don't hesitate to reach out. There's no reason that this sort of thing should be a one-man project. So let me know what you think, feel free to touch base any time, and check out the website for more.

Ryan

Ryan
Paramedic & Nurse
Managing Member, Rykerr Medical LLC

RYKERRMEDICAL.COM

References

The ARDS Network (2000). Ventilation with lower tidal volumes as compared with traditional tidal volumes for acute lung injury and the acute respiratory distress syndrome. *The New England Journal of Medicine, 342*(18).
Retrieved from https://www.nejm.org/doi/full/10.1056/NEJM200005043421801

Alexander, D. (2016). Approach to tachycardia in the ED setting. *emDocs.*
Retrieved from http://www.emdocs.net/approach-tachypnea-ed-setting/

Arjo (2020). *RotoProne: A Comprehensive System that Helps Simplify Prone Therapy.*
Retrieved from https://www.arjo.com/en-us/products/medical-beds/critical-care/rotoprone/

Ashworth, L. et al. (2018). Clinical management of pressure control ventilation: An algorithmic method of patient ventilatory management to address "forgotten but important variables." *Journal of Critical Care, 43*, 169-183. doi: https://doi.org/10.1016/j.jcrc.2017.08.046

Azizov, U. (2017). *Cardiovascular Changes with Ventilation.* [Video].
Retrieved from https://www.youtube.com/watch?v=rXZxDma9s5s

Banzett, R. B., Similowski, T., & Brown, R. (2013). Addressing respiratory discomfort in the ventilated patient. *Principles and Practices of Mechanical Ventilation*, 3rd ed. McGraw-Hill.
Retrieved from https://accessanesthesiology.mhmedical.com/content.aspx?bookid=520&sectionid=41692302#57079099

Bauer, E. (2016a). BiPAP: Do you understand absolute versus additive. *FlightBridgeED.* [Podcast].
Retrieved from https://www.flightbridgeed.com/index.php/the-flightbridgeed-podcast/2-flightbridgeed-podcast/88-bipap-do-you-understand-absolute-versus-additive

Bauer, E. (2016b). Driving pressure. *FlightBridgeED.* [Podcast].
Retrieved from https://www.flightbridgeed.com/index.php/the-flightbridgeed-podcast/2-flightbridgeed-podcast/189-driving-pressure

Bauer, E. (2016c). Henry's Law – fixing hypoxia? *FlightBridgeED.*
Retrieved from https://www.flightbridgeed.com/index.php/blogs/blogs-view/10-artcles/130-henry-s-law-fixing-hypoxia-1

Bauer, E. (2018). *Ventilator Management: A Pre-Hospital Perspective*, 2nd ed. FlightBridgeED; Scottsville, KY

Bauer, E. (2015). Ventilator strategy: Hypotension. *FlightBridgeED.* [Podcast]. Retrieved from https://www.flightbridgeed.com/index.php/the-flightbridgeed-podcast/2-flightbridgeed-podcast/56-ventilator-strategy-hypotension

Betts, J. G. et al. (2013). *Anatomy and Physiology.* Houston, TX: OpenStax. Retrieved from https://openstax.org/books/anatomy-and-physiology/pages/1-introduction

Bloomfield, R., Noble, D. W., & Sudlow, A. (2015). Prone position for acute respiratory failure in adults. *Cochrane Database of Systematic Reviews.* doi: https://doi.org/10.1002/14651858.CD008095.pub2

Boon, M. & Boon, B. (2018). A world upside down: Transporting prone. *Heavy Lies the Helmet.* [Podcast]. Retrieved from https://heavyliesthehelmet.com/2018/03/17/017/

Briggs, B. & Freese, J. (2018). Patient's elevated airway pressure puzzles providers. *Journal of Emergency Medical Services.* Retrieved from https://www.jems.com/2018/11/28/patient-s-elevated-airway-pressure-puzzles-providers/

Bugedo, G., Retamal, J., & Alejandro, B. (2017). Driving pressure: A marker of severity, a safety limit, or a goal for mechanical ventilation? *Critical Care, 21*(199). doi:10.1186/s13054-017-1779-x. Retrieved from https://ccforum.biomedcentral.com/articles/10.1186/s13054-017-1779-x#citeas

Carter, R., Tiep, B., & Boatright, D. (2010). Oxygen delivery and acid-base balance. *RTMagazine.com.* Retrieved from https://www.rtmagazine.com/disorders-diseases/chronic-pulmonary-disorders/chronic-diseases/oxygen-delivery-and-acid-base-balance/

Cassone, M., Cocciolone, A., & Meinychuk, E. (2019). Your first shift in the unit: Demystifying ventilator alarms. *EM Resident.* Retrieved from https://www.emra.org/emresident/article/demystifying_ventilator_alarms/

Chambers, N. A. et al. (2017). Cuffed vs. uncuffed tracheal tubes in children: A randomised controlled trial comparing leak, tidal volume and complications. *Anaesthesia, 73*(2), 160-168. doi: https://doi.org/10.1111/anae.14113

Chatburn, R. L., El-Khatib, M., & Mireles-Cabodevila, E. (2014). A taxonomy for mechanical ventilation: 10 fundamental maxims. *Respiratory Care, 59*(11), 1747-1763. doi: https://doi.org/10.4187/respcare.03057

Chatburn, R. L. & Mireles-Cabodevila., E. (2013). Basic principles of ventilator design. *Principles and Practices of Mechanical Ventilation*, 3rd ed. McGraw-Hill. Retrieved from https://accessanesthesiology.mhmedical.com/content.aspx?sectionid=41692239&bookid=520#57061229

Chemtob, R. A. & Moller-Sorenson, H. (2018). Peripheral measurements of venous oxygen saturation and lactate as a less invasive alternative for hemodynamic monitoring. *Scandinavian Journal of Resuscitation and Emergency Medicine, 26*(65). doi: 10.1186/s13049-018-0537-7. Retrieved from https://www.ncbi.nlm.nih.gov/pmc/articles/PMC6131814/

Chiefetz, I. M. (2014). Cardiorespiratory interactions: The relationship between mechanical ventilation and hemodynamics. *Respiratory Care, 54*(12), 1937-1945. doi: https://doi.org/10.4187/respcare.03486

Claire, et al. (2019). Lung recruitment maneuver. *WikiEM.* Retrieved from https://wikem.org/wiki/Lung_recruitment_maneuver

Coruh, B. & Luks, A. (2014). Positive end-expiratory pressure. When more may not be better. *Annals of American Thoracic Society, 11*(8), 1327-1331. doi: 10.1513/AnnalsATS.201404-151CC. Retrieved from https://www.atsjournals.org/doi/full/10.1513/AnnalsATS.201404-151CC#readcube-epdf

Clinical Analysis Management (2009). *CRASH Course*. [Video series]. Reviewed December 2019. Access to content at http://www.camanagement1.org/Clinical_Analysis/Why_Crash.html

Critical Care Cardiff (2017). *Turning Patient from Supine to Prone.* [Video]. Retrieved from https://www.youtube.com/watch?v=Cwu8zMYppis

Critical Care & Major Trauma Network (2015). *Prone Position 1.* [Video]. Retrieved from https://www.youtube.com/watch?v=bE4mmGdjA5I

Davies, J. D., Senussi, M. H., & Mireles-Cabodevila, E. (2016). Should a tidal volume of 6ml/kg be used in all patients? *Respiratory Care, 61*(6), 774-790. doi: https://doi.org/10.4187/respcare.04651

Desai, R. (2012). Oxygen movement from alveoli to capillaries. *Khan Academy.* [Video]. Retrieved from https://www.khanacademy.org/science/health-and-medicine/respiratory-system/gas-exchange-jv/v/oxygen-movement-from-alveoli-to-capillaries

Dhand, R. (2017). How should aerosols be delivered during invasive mechanical ventilation? *Respiratory Care, 61*(10), 1343-1367. doi: 10.4187/respcare.05803. Retrieved from http://rc.rcjournal.com/content/respcare/early/2017/09/05/respcare.05803.full.pdf

Dunham-Snary, K. et al. (2017). Hypoxic pulmonary vasoconstriction: From molecular mechanisms to medicine. *Chest, 151*(1), 181-192. doi: 10.1016/j.chest.2016.09.001. Retrieved from https://www.ncbi.nlm.nih.gov/pmc/articles/PMC5310129/

Dunphy, A. (2012). *Absorption Atelectasis.* [Video]. Retrieved from https://www.youtube.com/watch?v=m-d2IQC-sbM

Farkas, J. (2017). PulmCrit – APRV: Resurrection of the open-lung strategy? *EMCrit.* Retrieved from https://emcrit.org/pulmcrit/aprv/

Farkas, J. (2016). PulmCrit - Top 10 reasons pulse oximetry beats ABG for assessing oxygenation. *EMCrit.* Retrieved from https://emcrit.org/pulmcrit/pulse-oximetry/

Felix, N. S. et al. (2019). Gradually increasing tidal volume may mitigate experimental lung injury in rats. *Critical Care Medicine, 130*, 767-777. doi: https://doi.org/10.1097/ALN.0000000000002630

Flowers, P. et al. (2019). *Chemistry: Atoms first* (2nd ed.). Houston, TX: OpenStax. Retrieved from https://openstax.org/books/chemistry-atoms-first-2e/pages/1-introduction

Foster, T. & Grasso, S. (2014). Winter's formula. *Med School Made Easy.* [Video]. Retrieved from https://www.youtube.com/watch?v=nq0xSUJJf-4

Frakes, M. (2007). Ventilation modes and monitoring. *RTMagazine.com.* Retrieved from https://www.rtmagazine.com/products-treatment/diagnostics-testing/testing/ventilation-modes-and-monitoring/

George, J. (2015). Pneumonia vs. pneumonitis. *Khan Academy.* [Video]. Retrieved from https://www.khanacademy.org/science/health-and-medicine/respiratory-system-diseases/pneumonia/v/pneumonia-vs-pneumonitis

Ghamloush, M. & Hill, N. S. (2013). Synchronized intermittent mandatory ventilation: Time to send this workhorse out to pasture. *Respiratory Care, 58*(11), 1992-1994. doi: https://doi.org/10.4187/respcare.02880

Gillies, D. et al. (2017). Heat and moisture exchangers versus heated humidifiers for mechanically ventilated adults and children (review). *Cochrane Database of Systematic Reviews, 9.* doi: 1002/14651858.CD004711.pub3. Retrieved from https://www.cochranelibrary.com/cdsr/doi/10.1002/14651858.CD004711.pub3/epdf/full

Godoy, D. A. et al. (2017). Hyperventilation therapy for control of posttraumatic intracranial hypertension. *Frontiers in Neurology, 8*(250). doi: 10.3389/fneur.2017.00250. Retrieved from https://www.ncbi.nlm.nih.gov/pmc/articles/PMC5511895/

Goligher, E. C. (2017). Synchrony and the art of mechanical ventilation. *Anesthesiology, 127*(6), 915-917. doi: https://doi.org/10.1097/ALN.0000000000001921

Gonzales, J., Russian, C. J., & Henry, N. (2012). A review of waveform patterns for mechanically ventilated patients: Constant flow versus decelerating-flow waveform patterns. *RTMagazine.com.* Retrieved from https://www.rtmagazine.com/disorders-diseases/chronic-pulmonary-disorders/copd/a-review-of-waveform-patterns-for-mechanically-ventilated-patients-constant-flow-versus-decelerating-flow-waveform-patterns/

Graves, L. et al. (2014). A comparison of actual to estimated weights in Australian children attending a tertiary children's' hospital, using the original and updated APLS, Luscombe and Owens, Best Guess formulae and the Broselow tape. *Resuscitation, 85*(3), 392-396. doi: https://doi.org/10.1016/j.resuscitation.2013.11.024

Grune, J., Tabuchi, A., & Kuebler, W. M. (2019). Alveolar dynamics during mechanical ventilation in the healthy and injured lung. *Intensive Care Medicine Experimental, 7*(34). doi: 10.1186/s40635-019-0226-5. Retrieved from https://www.ncbi.nlm.nih.gov/pmc/articles/PMC6658629/?report=classic

Hartland, B. L., Newell, T. J., & Damico, N. (2015). Alveolar recruitment maneuvers under general anesthesia: A systematic review of the literature. *Respiratory Care, 60*(4), 609-620. doi: https://doi.org/10.4187/respcare.03488

Hill, J. (2019). Is a bag enough? *Taming the SRU.* Retrieved from http://www.tamingthesru.com/blog/2019/9/7/is-a-bag-enough

Henderson, W. R. et al. (2014). Does prone positioning improve oxygenation and reduce mortality in patients with acute respiratory distress syndrome? *Canadian Respiratory Journal, 21*(4), 213-215. doi: 10.1155/2014/472136.
Retrieved from https://www.ncbi.nlm.nih.gov/pmc/articles/PMC4173887/

Hess, D. R. (2015). Recruitment maneuvers and PEEP titration. *Respiratory Care, 60*(11), 1688-1704. doi: https://doi.org/10.4187/respcare.04409

Hess, D. R. (2014). Respiratory mechanics in mechanically ventilated patients. *Respiratory Care, 59*(11), 1773-1794. doi: 10.4187/respcare.03410.
Retrieved from http://rc.rcjournal.com/content/respcare/early/2014/10/21/respcare.03410.full.pdf

Hess, D. R. (2005). Ventilator waveforms and the physiology of pressure support ventilation. *Respiratory Care, 50*(2), 166-186. Retrieved from http://rc.rcjournal.com/content/50/2/166/tab-pdf

Hinkson, C. R. et al. (2006). The effects of apparatus dead space on $PaCO_2$ in patients receiving lung-protective ventilation. *Respiratory Care, 51*(10), 1140-1144.
Retrieved from http://www.rcjournal.com/contents/10.06/10.06.1140.pdf

Hodgson, C. et al. (2016). Recruitment manoeuvres for adults with acute respiratory distress syndrome receiving mechanical ventilation. *Cochrane Database of Systematic Reviews.* doi: https://doi.org/10.1002/14651858.CD006667.pub3

Hospital Direct (2017). *ProTurn - Patient Proning Solved - Supine to Prone - Hospital Direct Acute.* [Video]. Retrieved from https://www.youtube.com/watch?v=xprH8_8GjBg

Iyer, V. & Holets, S. (2016). Ventilator waveforms: Basic interpretation and analysis. *Thoracic.org.* [PowerPoint Presentation]. Retrieved from https://www.thoracic.org/professionals/clinical-resources/critical-care/clinical-education/mechanical-ventilation/ventilator-waveform-analysis.php

Johnston, R. (2015). Anatomic dead space. *PFT Blog.* Retrieved from https://www.pftforum.com/blog/anatomic-dead-space/

Johnston, R. (2017). What does an inverse I:E ratio during exercise mean? *PFT Blog.* Retrieved from https://www.pftforum.com/blog/what-does-an-inverse-ie-ratio-during-exercise-mean/

Kacmarek, R. M. & Branson, R. D. (2016). Should intermittent mandatory ventilation be abolished? *Respiratory Care, 61*(6), 854-866. doi: https://doi.org/10.4187/respcare.04887

Kallet, R. H. & Branson, R. D. (2016). Should oxygen therapy be tightly regulated to minimize hyperoxia in critically ill patients? *Respiratory Care, 61*(6), 801-817. Retrieved from http://rc.rcjournal.com/content/respcare/61/6/801.full.pdf

Kindig, M. et al. (2019). A tale of two tapes: Broselow-Luten tapes, 2011 vs. 2017. *Journal of Emergency Medical Services*. Retrieved from https://www.jems.com/2019/04/29/a-tale-of-two-tapes-broselow-luten-tapes-2011-vs-2017/

Kneyber, M. et al. (2017). Recommendations for mechanical ventilation of critically ill children from the Paediatric Mechanical Ventilation Consensus Conference (PEMVECC). *Intensive Care Medicine, 43*(12), 1764-80. doi: 10.1007/s00134-017-4920-z. Retrieved from https://www.ncbi.nlm.nih.gov/pmc/articles/PMC5717127/

Koulouras, V. et al. (2016). Efficacy of prone position in acute respiratory distress syndrome patients: A pathophysiology-based review. *World Journal of Critical Care Medicine, 5*(2), 121-136. doi: 10.5492/wjccm.v5.i2.121. Retrieved from https://www.ncbi.nlm.nih.gov/pmc/articles/PMC4848155/#B23&#8221

Kuhn, B. T., et al. (2016). Management of mechanical ventilation in decompensated heart failure. *Journal of Cardiovascular Development and Disease, 3*(4), 33. doi: 10.3390/jcdd3040033. Retrieved from https://www.ncbi.nlm.nih.gov/pmc/articles/PMC5715720/

Kumar, A. J. (2015). Synchronized intermittent mandatory ventilation (SIMV). *EMmedonline.* Retrieved from https://emmedonline.com/airway/simv

Lauria, M., Norii, T., & Soneru, C. (2019). Fixing a cuff leak: Learning to improvise with airway problems. *EMResident.* Retrieved from https://www.emra.org/emresident/article/cuff-leak/

Lodeserto, F. (2018). Simplifying mechanical ventilation. *RebelEM.* [Article Series]. First article retrieved from https://rebelem.com/simplifying-mechanical-ventilation-part/

LoMauro, A. & Aliverti, A. (2015). Respiratory physiology in pregnancy: Physiology masterclass. *Breathe, 11*(4), 297-301. doi: 10.1183/20734735.008615. Retrieved from https://www.ncbi.nlm.nih.gov/pmc/articles/PMC4818213/

Luecke, T. & Pelosi, P. (2005). Clinical review: Positive end-expiratory pressure and cardiac output. *Critical Care, 9*(6), 607-621. doi: 10.1186/cc3877. Retrieved from https://www.ncbi.nlm.nih.gov/pmc/articles/PMC1414045/

Lumb, A. B. & Slinger, P. (2015). Hypoxic pulmonary vasoconstriction: Physiology and anesthetic implications. *Anesthesiology, 122*(4), 932-946. doi: https://doi.org/10.1097/ALN.0000000000000569

Macintyre, N. R. (2014). Tissue hypoxia: Implications for the respiratory clinician. *Respiratory Care, 59*(10) 1590-1596. doi: https://doi.org/10.4187/respcare.03357

Maher, R. (2019). Mechanical ventilation- 52: Pressure regulated volume control (PRVC) part 1. *Hospitalista.* [Video]. Retrieved from https://www.youtube.com/watch?v=X0VpueL6Chk

Mahmood, S. S. & Pinsky, M. R. (2018). Heart-lung interactions during mechanical ventilation: The basics. *Annals of Translational Medicine, 6*(18). doi: 10.21037/atm.2018.04.29. Retrieved from https://www.ncbi.nlm.nih.gov/pmc/articles/PMC6186561/pdf/atm-06-18-349.pdf

Mannarino, I. (2014). Shock – diagnosis and treatment. *Khan Academy.* [Video]. Retrieved from https://www.khanacademy.org/science/health-and-medicine/circulatory-system-diseases/shock/v/shock-oxygen-delivery-and-metabolism

Mason, M. J. (2019). Respiratory physiology. *Hippomedics.* [Video Series]. Retrieved from https://www.youtube.com/playlist?list=PLKbsytZxJw7_ObYvaAtmrzbFDUIzJvdU2

Mauri, T. et al. (2017). Spontaneous breathing: A double-edged sword to handle with care. *Annals of Translational Medicine, 5*(14). doi: 10.21037/atm.2017.06.55. Retrieved from https://www.ncbi.nlm.nih.gov/pmc/articles/PMC5537122/

Meeks, C. (2018). Final decision: Commentary on volume vs. pressure. *Mind Body Medic.* [Podcast]. Retrieved from https://flightbridgeed.com/index.php/mindbodymedic-podcast/11-mindbodymedicpodcast/324-final-decision-commentary-on-volume-vs-pressure

Mellick, L. (2014). *Endotracheal Tube Change Over a Bougie*. [Video]. Retrieved from https://www.youtube.com/watch?v=ERnJY9p-BfY

Metz, A. (2016a). *Recruitment maneuver.* [Video]. Retrieved from https://www.youtube.com/watch?v=w0bJLStW6Zs

Metz, A. (2016b). *Stepwise recruitment maneuver.* [Video]. Retrieved from https://www.youtube.com/watch?v=QCsBMMsUsZE

Mojoli, F., et al. (2015). Automatic monitoring of plateau and driving pressure during pressure and volume controlled ventilation. *Intensive Care Medicine Experimental, 3*(Suppl 1), A998. doi:10.1186/2197-425X-3-S1-A998. Retrieved from https://www.ncbi.nlm.nih.gov/pmc/articles/PMC4798316/pdf/40635_2015_Article_1137.pdf

Mojoli, F. (2017). Ultrasound-guided mechanical ventilation. *ICU Practice & Management, 17* (3), 186-189. Retrieved from https://healthmanagement.org/c/icu/issuearticle/ultrasound-guided-mechanical-ventilation

Murias, G., Blanch, L., & Lucangelo, U. (2014). The physiology of ventilation. *Respiratory Care, 59*(11), 1795-1807. doi: https://doi.org/10.4187/respcare.03377

Murphy, Z, (2017a). Regulation of breathing: Factors influencing rate and depth | Part 3. *Ninja Nerd Science.* [Video]. Retrieved from https://www.youtube.com/watch?v=gSVtW1HcV3c&list=PLTF9h-T1TcJjdJppplKVsgPWNQ_beElaG&index=19&t=0s

Murphy, Z. (2017b). Types of hypoxia: Hypoxic | Anemic | Stagnant | Histotoxic. *Ninja Nerd Science.* [Video]. Retrieved from https://www.youtube.com/watch?v=RlpBOOb8KkU

Nagler, J. & Chiefetz, I. M. (2019). Initiating mechanical ventilation in children. *UpToDate.* Retrieved from https://www.uptodate.com/contents/initiating-mechanical-ventilation-in-children

Naik, B. I., Lynch, C., & Durbin, C. G. (2015). Variability in mechanical ventilation: What's all the noise about? *Respiratory Care, 60*(8), 1203-1210. doi: https://doi.org/10.4187/respcare.03794

Nargis, W. et al (2015). Comparison of values of traditionally measured venous bicarbonate with calculated arterial bicarbonate in intensive care unit patients of a hospital in a third-world country. *Nigerian Medical Journal, 55*(4), 285-288. doi: 10.4103/0300-1652.137186.
Retrieved from https://www.ncbi.nlm.nih.gov/pmc/articles/PMC4124539/

NHLBI ARDS Network (2004). Higher versus lower Positive End-Expiratory Pressures in patients with the Acute Respiratory Distress Syndrome. *New England Journal of Medicine, 351*, 327-336. doi: 10.1056/NEJMoa032193.
Retrieved from https://www.nejm.org/doi/full/10.1056/NEJMoa032193

Nickson, C. (2019a). High airway and alveolar pressures. *Life in the Fast Lane.* Retrieved from https://litfl.com/high-airway-and-alveolar-pressures/

Nickson, C. (2019b). Open lung approach to ventilation. *Life in the Fast Lane.* Retrieved from https://litfl.com/open-lung-approach-to-ventilation/

Ochs, M. et al. (2003). The number of alveoli in the human lung. *American Journal of Respiratory and Critical Care Medicine, 169*(1). doi: https://doi.org/10.1164/rccm.200308-1107OC

Ollie (2015). Principles of mechanical ventilation 14: SIMV. *Respiratory Review.* [Video]. Retrieved from https://www.youtube.com/watch?v=RsV31UlH3yU

Olveira, V. M., et al. (2017). Safe prone checklist: construction and implementation of a tool for performing the prone maneuver. *Revista Brasileira de Terapia Intensiva, 29*(2), 131-141. doi: 10.5935/0103-507X.20170023. Retrieved from https://www.ncbi.nlm.nih.gov/pmc/articles/PMC5496747/#r3

Patel, H. & Bhardwaj, A. (2018). Physiology, respiratory quotient. *Stat Pearls.* Treasure Island, FL: StatPearls Publishing. Retrieved from https://www.ncbi.nlm.nih.gov/books/NBK531494/

Patel, S. B. & Kress, J. P. (2011). Sedation and analgesia in the mechanically ventilated patient. *American Journal of Respiratory and Critical Care Medicine, 185*(5). doi: https://doi.org/10.1164/rccm.201102-0273CI

Perlman, C. E., Lederer, D. J., & Bhattacharya, J. (2010). Micromechanics of alveolar edema. *American Journal of Respiratory Cell and Molecular Biology, 44*(1), 34-39. doi: 10.1165/rcmb.2009-0005OC. Retrieved from https://www.ncbi.nlm.nih.gov/pmc/articles/PMC3028256/

Prost, A. (2011). *High Frequency Oscillation Ventilation.* [Video]. Retrieved from https://www.youtube.com/watch?v=l-0pm84AA4o

Pruitt, W. (2007). Permissive hypercapnia. *RTMagazine.com.* Retrieved from https://www.rtmagazine.com/disorders-diseases/chronic-pulmonary-disorders/asthma/permissive-hypercapnia/

Radermacher, P., Maggiore, S. M., & Mercat, A. (2017). Fifty years of research in ARDS: Gas exchange in Acute Respiratory Distress Syndrome. *American Journal of Respiratory and Critical Care Medicine, 196*(8), 964-984. doi: : 10.1164/rccm.201610-2156SO. Retrieved from https://www.atsjournals.org/doi/10.1164/rccm.201610-2156SO

Ragaller, M. & Richter, T. (2010). Acute lung injury and acute respiratory distress syndrome. *Journal of Emergencies, Trauma, and Shock, 3*(1), 43-51. doi: 10.4103/0974-2700.58663. Retrieved from https://www.ncbi.nlm.nih.gov/pmc/articles/PMC2823143/

Reading, J. (2016). Understanding the relationship between oxygen flow rate and FiO_2. *Ausmed.* Retrieved from https://www.ausmed.com/cpd/articles/oxygen-flow-rate-and-fio2

Rezaie, S. (2018). Vent management in the crashing patient with Haney Mallemat. *RebelEM.* Retrieved from https://rebelem.com/rebel-cast-ep-46b-vent-management-crashing-patient-haney-mallemat/

Robertson, H. T. (2015). Dead space: The physiology of wasted ventilation. *European Respiratory Journal, 45*, 1704-1716. doi: 10.1183/09031936.50137614. Retrieved from https://erj.ersjournals.com/content/46/4/1226

Sahetya, S. K., Manceba, J., & Brower, R. G. (2017). Fifty years of research in ARDS: Vt selection in Acute Respiratory Distress Syndrome. *American Journal of Respiratory and Critical Care Medicine, 196*(12). doi: https://doi.org/10.1164/rccm.201708-1629CI.

ScyMed (2018). *MediCalc: Pulmonary.* Retrieved from http://www.scymed.com/en/smnxpr/smnxpr.htm#prkao000

Silverston, P. (2016). Pulse oximetry: Uses and limitations. *Geeky Medics.* Retrieved from https://geekymedics.com/pulse-oximetry/

Siobal, M. A. (2016). Monitoring exhaled carbon dioxide. *Respiratory Care, 61*(10), 1397-1416. doi: 10.4187/respcare.04919. Retrieved from http://rc.rcjournal.com/content/respcare/early/2016/09/06/respcare.04919.full.pdf

Smith, N. (2004). Respiratory: ABG interpretation. *5 Minute Medicine.* [Video]. Retrieved from https://www.youtube.com/watch?v=14FTCPcx80I

Speller, J. (2018). Gas exchange. *TeachMe Physiology.* Retrieved from https://teachmephysiology.com/respiratory-system/gas-exchange/gas-exchange/

Spooner, A. J. et al. (2014). Head-of-bed elevation improves end-expiratory lung volumes in mechanically ventilated subjects: a prospective observational study. *Respiratory Care, 59*(10), 1583-1589. Retrieved from http://rc.rcjournal.com/content/respcare/59/10/1583.full.pdf

Stather, D. R. & Stewart, T. E. (2005). Clinical review: Mechanical ventilation in severe asthma. *Critical Care, 9*(6), 581-587. doi: 10.1186/cc3733. Retrieved from https://www.ncbi.nlm.nih.gov/pmc/articles/PMC1414026/

Strong, E. (2014). ABG interpretation. *Strong Medicine.* [Video Series]. Retrieved from https://www.youtube.com/playlist?list=PLFDCF820E88FC83ED

Strong, E. (2013). Physiologic consequences (mechanical ventilation - lecture 10). *Strong Medicine.* [Video]. Retrieved from https://www.youtube.com/watch?v=plcrzGTOBmw

Swaminathan, A. (2015). Is too much supplemental O_2 harmful in COPD exacerbations? *RebelEM.* Retrieved from https://rebelem.com/is-too-much-supplemental-o2-harmful-in-copd-exacerbations/

Tennyson, J. et al. (2016). Endotracheal tube cuff pressures in patients intubated prior to helicopter EMS transport. *Western Journal of Emergency Medicine, 17*(6), 721-725. doi: 10.5811/westjem.2016.8.30639. Retrieved from https://escholarship.org/uc/item/72p7845j

Thomas, V. K. & Abraham, S. V. (2018). Adding an "R" in the "DOPE" mnemonic for ventilator troubleshooting. *Indian Journal of Critical Care Medicine, 22*(5), 388. doi: 10.4103/ijccm.IJCCM_501_17. Retrieved from https://www.ncbi.nlm.nih.gov/pmc/articles/PMC5971655/

Tobin, M. J. et al. (2010). Ventilator-induced respiratory muscle weakness. *Annals of Internal Medicine, 153*(4), 240-245. doi: 10.1059/0003-4819-153-4-201008170-00006. Retrieved from https://www.ncbi.nlm.nih.gov/pmc/articles/PMC2924757/

Trainor, A. et al (2019). Mechanical ventilation 101: Compliance and resistance. *American Thoracic Society.* [Video]. Retrieved from https://www.thoracic.org/professionals/clinical-resources/video-lecture-series/mechanical-ventilation/mechanical-ventilation-101-resistance-and-compliance.php

van der Zee, P. & Gommers, D. (2019). Recruitment maneuvers and higher PEEP, the so-called open lung concept, in patients with ARDS. *Critical Care, 23*(73). doi: https://doi.org/10.1186/s13054-019-2365-1

Weingart, S. (2016a). Driving pressure with Dr. Roy Brower. *EMCrit.* [Podcast]. Retrieved from https://emcrit.org/emcrit/driving-pressure/

Weingart, S. (2009). Laryngoscope as a murder weapon (LAMW) series – ventilatory kills – intubating the patient with severe metabolic acidosis. *EMCrit.* [Podcast]. Retrieved from https://emcrit.org/emcrit/tube-severe-acidosis/

Weingart, S. (2016b). Managing initial mechanical ventilation in the emergency department. *Annals of Emergency Medicine*.
Retrieved from https://emcrit.org/wp-content/uploads/2010/05/Managing-Initial-Vent-ED.pdf

Weingart, S, (2011). Origins of the dope mnemonic. *EMCrit.*
Retrieved from https://emcrit.org/emcrit/origins-of-the-dope-mnemonic/

Weingart, S. (2010). Spinning dials: how to dominate the vent. *EMCrit.* [Podcast Series].
Retrieved from: https://emcrit.org/emcrit/vent-part-1/

Weingart, S. (2019). Vent alarms = code blue. *EMCrit.* [Podcast].
Retrieved from https://emcrit.org/emcrit/vent-alarms/

Wheeler, D. S., Wong, H. R., & Shanley, T. P. (2008). Chapter 6: Mechanical ventilation. *The Respiratory Tract in Pediatric Illness & Injury.* Springer Science & Business Media.
Retrieved from https://books.google.com/books?id=1o1iUQUCSwgC&printsec=frontcover&source=gbs_ge_summary_r&cad=0#v=onepage&q&f=false

Wilkes, A. R. (2011a). Heat and moisture exchangers and breathing system filters: Their use in anesthesia and intensive care. Part 1 – history, principles and efficiency. *Anesthesia, 66*, 31-39. doi: 10.1111/j.1365-2044.2010.06563.x.
Retrieved from https://onlinelibrary.wiley.com/doi/pdf/10.1111/j.1365-2044.2010.06563.x

Wilkes, A. R. (2011b). Heat and moisture exchangers and breathing system filters: Their use in anesthesia and intensive care. Part 2 – practical use, including problems, and their use with paediatric patients. *Anesthesia, 66*, 40-51. doi: 10.1111/j.1365-2044.2010.06564.x.
Retrieved from https://onlinelibrary.wiley.com/doi/pdf/10.1111/j.1365-2044.2010.06564.x

Wingfield, W. (2012a). High risk OB/ GYN. *The Ace Prep Course.* [Video].
Retrieved from https://www.theresqshop.com/category-s/101.htm

Wingfield, W. (2012b). Pulmonary disease and ventilators. *The Ace Prep Course.* [Video].
Retrieved from https://www.theresqshop.com/category-s/101.htm

Woodruff, D. W. (2007). Six steps to ABG analysis. *Nursing Critical Care, 2*(2), 48-52. doi: 10.1097/01.CCN.0000264040.77759.bf. Retrieved from https://journals.lww.com/nursingcriticalcare/fulltext/2007/03000/six_steps_to_abg_analysis.13.aspx

Wright, B. J. (2014). Lung-protective ventilation strategies and adjunctive treatments for the emergency medicine patient with acute respiratory failure. *Emergency Medicine Clinics of North America, 32*(4), 871-887. doi: https://doi.org/10.1016/j.emc.2014.07.012

Writing Group for the PReVENT Investigators (2018). Effect of a low vs intermediate tidal volume on ventilator-free days in intensive care patients without ARDS: A randomized clinical trial. *Journal of the American Medical Association, 320*(18), 1872-1880. doi: 10.1001/jama.2018.14280. Retrieved from https://jamanetwork.com/journals/jama/fullarticle/2710774

Yartsev, A. (2019). Respiratory system. [Section in website]. *Deranged Physiology.* Retrieved from https://derangedphysiology.com/main/cicm-primary-exam/required-reading/respiratory-system

Made in United States
North Haven, CT
05 November 2026

21763952R00111